D0218867

The Perceptual World

The Perceptual World

. . .

READINGS FROM
SCIENTIFIC AMERICAN MAGAZINE

Edited by

Irvin Rock
University of California at Berkeley

W. H. FREEMAN AND COMPANY
New York

Some of the SCIENTIFIC AMERICAN articles in *The Perceptual World* are available as separate Offprints. For a complete list of articles now available as Offprints, write to Product Manager, Marketing Department, W. H. Freeman and Company, 41 Madison Avenue, New York, New York 10010.

Library of Congress Cataloging-in-Publication Data

The perceptual world: readings from Scientific American
    magazine / edited by Irvin Rock.
       p.   cm.
    Includes bibliographical references.
    ISBN 0-7167-2068-X
    1. Vision. 2. Visual perception. I. Rock, Irvin.
II. Scientific American.
QP475.P38 1990   89-17082
152.14--dc20   CIP

Copyright © 1974, 1976, 1977, 1979, 1980, 1984, 1986, 1988 by Scientific American, Inc.

Copyright © 1990 by W. H. Freeman and Company

No part of this book may be reproduced by any mechanical, photographic, or electronic process, or in the form of a phonographic recording, nor may it be stored in a retrieval system, transmitted, or otherwise copied for public or private use, without written permission from the publisher.

Printed in the United States of America

1 2 3 4 5 6 7 8 9 0 RRD 89

CONTENTS

SECTION IV: OBJECT AND EVENT PERCEPTION

SECTION V: ILLUSORY PHENOMENA

SECTION VI: PERCEPTION AND IMAGERY

Note on cross-references to SCIENTIFIC AMERICAN *articles:* Articles included in this book are referred to by chapter number and title; articles not included in this book but available as Offprints are referred to by title, date of publication and Offprint number; articles not in this book and not available as Offprints are referred to by title and date of publication.

Editorial changes were at times required in the adaptation of articles to the format of the Reader; these changes are in brackets.

Introduction

In the last 20 years the fields of sensory and perceptual processes have mushroomed into major subdivisions of psychology and neurophysiology. The articles from SCIENTIFIC AMERICAN presented here represent important developments during this period; indeed, some of the research described was done only in the last few years. The topics range from neurophysiological discoveries concerning specific brain mechanisms to experiments on mental imagery and its relationship to perception. The reader will see from the introductory comments in each article that, in most cases, the authors were grappling with well-known perceptual problems—why, for example, in a geometrical illusion figure, one line looks longer than another of equivalent length. In some cases, however, new phenomena or facts have been discovered—for example, the columns in the visual cortex that alternately represent the dominant and nondominant eyes of the observer, or the phenomenon of subjective contours, or aftereffects in which color and contour orientation are linked to one another. Once discovered, these facts themselves have become the subject of inquiry.

The first two chapters cover work on brain mechanisms. Chapter 1, "Brain Mechanisms of Vision," describes the landmark discoveries made by the authors David H. Hubel and Torsten N. Wiesel in 1959, for which they later received the Nobel Prize. They found that individual neurons at various levels in the visual nervous system will discharge rapidly ("fire") when a certain pattern of stimulation is present on an appropriate region of the retina of the eye. For example, in response to a bar or edge, a cell in the visual cortex will fire rapidly if and only if the image is in a certain orientation on the retina. Thus, one might say that the cell "detects" the presence of the bar pattern on the retina.

These findings represent an enormous stride forward in sensory physiology, although the precise function of these detector cells is still not known.

Chapter 2, "Negative Aftereffects in Visual Perception," by Olga E. Favreau and Michael C. Corballis refers to a broad class of effects in which one perceives something illusory as a result of what one had been looking at previously. The authors search for the brain mechanism underlying effects of this kind. Some such effects—for example, a color afterimage—have been known for a long time, but others are recent discoveries. The authors examine the plausible theory that aftereffects can be explained by the fatiguing of certain cells on the retina or deeper in the brain.

Important developments in our understanding of color and lightness vision are addressed next in Chapter 3, "The Retinex Theory of Color Vision," by Edwin H. Land, and Chapter 4, "The Perception of Surface Blacks and Whites," by Alan L. Gilchrist. Land, already famous for his development and manufacture of the camera that bears his name, is concerned here with the problem of the perception of chromatic colors, or hues. He presents an ingenious theory, supported by ingenious experiments, namely that each set of cone cells in the retina generates an achromatic image of the scene as viewed through the filter of its own photopigment. The color of any single surface is obtained by comparing its lightness within each of those three differing achromatic images.

Gilchrist's chapter is concerned with a problem that few people realize *is* a problem, namely, the perception of the shades of gray or white or black of a surface, referred to nowadays by the term *lightness*. The problem is this: What determines perceived lightness? It can't simply be the intensity of light the surface reflects to the eye, because its lightness will continue to look the same in almost any illumination. There is now agreement that the answer to this question bears in some way on the visual system picking up information about *ratios* of light intensity reflected from neighboring surfaces. Gilchrist shows that acquiring such ratio information is only the first step in a further sequence of events that requires integration of the changes of such ratios as well as making the distinction between adjacent edges that differ in reflectance from those that differ in illumination. Interestingly, Land's theory makes use of this notion of intensity ratios in explaining the computation of lightnesses underlying the perception of hues.

Over the last two decades the prevailing approach has been to explain perception and cognition by the information-processing model: data received by the sense organs are processed in a series of stages, each of which requires a certain amount of processing time. The field of artificial intelligence has sought to stimulate such information processing with the use of digital computers. In the case of perception, this approach has been referred to as "machine vision." In Chapter 5, "Vision by Man and Machine," we see a good example of this approach, as Tomaso Poggio and his co-workers try to determine how we achieve depth perception by retinal disparity (i.e., from the slightly different images the two eyes receive in viewing a scene). He describes an algorithm by which a computer, given the necessary pair of visual inputs, could indeed solve the problem.

Anne Treisman in Chapter 6, "Features and Objects in Visual Processing," grapples with the problem of whether the processing underlying perception is based on simultaneous (or "parallel") processing of all the elements in a scene or on sequential (or "serial") processing. In the former case, attention to each element obviously would not be possible (or necessary), whereas in the latter case, the very reason for serial processing might be that we must attend to each item. Her findings, making use of new methods that she and others have developed, suggest that the segregation of the scene into homogeneous regions is based on parallel processing of elements, provided that such segregation is accomplished with respect to single properties of such elements—for example, color—whereas the detection of an item or of regions based on the *combination* of properties—for example, both color and shape—requires serial processing, with attention to each item in turn.

The perception of objects and events is a traditional area of research, wherein the higher-level aspects of what we see are distinguished from the lower-level aspects, although no sharp dividing line exists between these levels. Such simple sensory qualities as hues or odors, for example, require no reference to objects. A property such as shape, size, motion or depth, however, is necessarily associated with an object or with relations among objects, and we generally cannot explain perception of such qualities by processes that occur in the sensory organ alone.

Chapter 7, "The Perception of Disoriented Figures," written by this author, deals with the problem of why shapes often look so different—and may not even be recognizable—when they are rotated or inverted. This fact is puzzling since other kinds of transformations that preserve the internal geometry of a figure do not affect its perceived shape, as when we enlarge or reduce it. The experiments I describe attempt to separate the effect of changing the image's orientation on the retina from that of changing the objects' orientation in the environment. The subject-observers are required to alter their orientation in a test wherein they view novel objects, after having seen them previously when both the observers and the objects were upright. In the test, the objects are sometimes upright in the environment and sometimes tilted in the way the observers are tilted. The results imply that the perceived shape of an object is in part a function of a frame of reference that we impose upon it.

In Chapter 8, "Perceiving Shape from Shading," Vilayanur S. Ramachandran sheds new light on a phenomenon known for some time by perception investigators. The location of shading within an object or in a picture of one will affect the object's perceived depth. Shading at the bottom of a region makes that region look like a mound, convexity or elevation; shadow at the top makes the same region look like a concavity, depression or hole. For this reason, inversion of such a picture will generally reverse the depth. The author explores the hypothesis that this effect is based on two "assumptions" the mind makes: that light comes from above and that there is only one such source of light for any given scene.

Then Ramachandran and Stuart M. Anstis in Chapter 9, "The Perception of Apparent Motion," explore the effect that underlies our perception of motion in moving pictures and television. A rapid series of still images yields a vivid impression of continuous movement. The authors focus on the problem of correspondence, how the mind knows which elements in successive views correspond to each other, a problem that can be made difficult in the laboratory by making the successive views ambiguous in this regard. They uncover new principles that correspond to features of the physical environment in which we have evolved: a tendency toward "assuming" inertia and the rigidity of objects.

Two chapters represent work in illusory phenomena. Gaetano Kanisza in Chapter 10 describes subjective contours, sometimes called illusory or cognitive contours. Although these effects were known for many years, with a few examples of them in print, they were paid little attention, perhaps because the examples were not striking. Kanisza's work, with his very powerful illustrations, opened a floodgate of interest in the effect. Not only are contours perceived at borders, where there are no physical differences in light intensity, but the figures that are seen also appear to be different from their backgrounds in lightness, mostly whiter in the figures in Kanisza's article. Barbara Gillam in Chapter 11 discusses the geometrical illusions that have for so long intrigued people. Most of the well-known illusions were first published in the last century and, despite countless later papers, there is still no accepted theory of any of them, let alone of all of them collectively. One favorite theory of many contemporary investigators is that these illusions result from the inappropriate attribution of depth to the patterns. That in turn yields constancy effects, so that, for example, a line in a drawing that appears farther away will appear longer than it would otherwise. (See "Visual Illusions," by Richard L. Gregory; SCIENTIFIC AMERICAN, November, 1968.) Gillam suggests that the illusory patterns *directly* yield size-constancy effects rather than first yielding depth cues that only then lead to constancy effects, and she presents some compelling new evidence and cogent arguments in support of her view.

The last chapter by Ronald A. Finke, "Mental Imagery and the Visual System," describes recent work on the relationship of perception to mental imagery. This is a topic of great interest to contemporary investigators. Mental images, obviously similar in certain respects to percepts, nevertheless require no stimulus input to a sense organ. But Finke and others have shown by ingenious experiments how one can go beyond this insight and explore the similarities between percepts and images. It appears not only that mental imagery is perceptionlike but,

more surprising, that perception can be affected by mental imagery.

For many readers, the chapters that follow will be comprehensible without further background, given the authors' clear discussions of the problems they address and the knowledge available at the time of their research. For those without any familiarity with the field of perception, I have endeavored to provide some background to the major issues here.

The Field of Perception

Most people are puzzled to learn that perception is an important discipline of psychology. They know that the eye is like a camera and that it takes a picture, albeit a continuous and moving one, of the scene. The picture is registered in the back of the eye. That "picture" is then transmitted by nerve fibers into the brain, where it is processed. The result is our subjective impression, or perception, of the scene, including the colors, shades, shapes, sizes and motions of the objects in it. To be sure, one would want to know more about the physiology of the registration of the "picture" on the retina of the eye and the transmission of it by neurons into the brain and the like, but aside from such neurophysiological questions, what kind of problems would lead to the emergence of a special field of inquiry called *perception*?

The analogy of eye to camera is a remarkably good one, as shown in Figure I.1, but only up to a point. In both the eye and the camera, light enters through a small opening, the size of which can vary to let in more or less light; in both cases, multiple rays of light from any given point in the scene are focused by a lens, the optical properties of which vary with the distance from which the rays emanate. Light is then projected onto the rear of the structure— the film in a camera, or the retina in the eye—and the image formed there is inverted top for bottom and reversed left for right. And in both cases both the intensity and wavelengths of the light emanating from each point in the scene are recorded when projected to the corresponding regions of the retina or film.

When such a retinal image, a faithful "picture" of the scene in many respects, is transmitted into the brain, what process accounts for our ensuing visual experience of the world? In other words, what is it that enables the seeing and interpretation of the image? Were there a little conscious person, or "homunculus," in the brain viewing that "picture," as

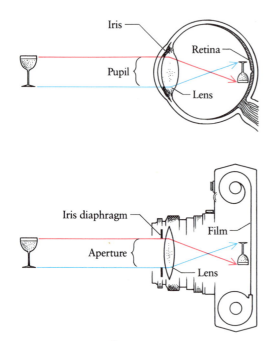

Figure I.1 SIMILARITY of eye and camera.

some philosophers through the centuries have suggested, the conscious visual experience of that "person" would explain perception. But virtually all modern philosophers and psychologists reject this kind of explanation. Among its other difficulties is that perception by this homunculus would then have to be explained, thus leading to an infinite regress of explanations.

Contemporary investigators argue instead that neither we nor homunculi in our heads *see* our retinal image; rather we perceive *on the basis of* the retinal image, that is, the image simply provides the first stage in our perception of the world. This emphasis incidentally clears up one puzzle of perception: why we perceive the world as upright despite the fact that the retinal image is upside down. Since no one is looking at the retinal image, its orientation is irrelevant. What matters is that it conveys the necessary spatial relationships about the world, which it does. As the Irish philosopher Bishop Berkeley noted almost three centuries ago, within the image, the feet are on the ground and the head is closer to the sky.

If there are no homunculi in the head, we must conclude that certain events going on in the brain

account for our visual perception. This simple step in reasoning is very important philosophically. It implies that our perception of the world is a construction of it. It forces us to realize that the physical world, which we assume exists independent of perception, should not be confused with our perception of that world.

The distinction between the physical world and the perceived world is further clarified by the distinction between physical properties of the world and the corresponding perceived properties. There are no colors such as red, blue and green in the physical world, only rays of light of varying wavelengths reflected from surfaces. There are no odors or tastes in the physical world, only certain chemical concentrations in the air or mouth. There are no sounds in the world, only vibrations created in the air. Colors, odors, tastes and sounds are the end result of the brain constructing such subjective sensations on the basis of the stimulation from the world impinging on a sense organ.

If perception is indeed a construction of the brain and mind, several questions arise. First, what is the level of the construction? Physicists tell us that the world consists of electromagnetic fields, atomic particles and the empty spaces that separate atomic nuclei from the charged particles that spin around them, but our perception of the world is not at this level. Rather, our perception is limited by the range of stimuli to which our senses are attuned.

Second, how faithful is our construction to reality? Why and how does it come about that the perceptual construction is a sufficiently accurate representation of the scene to enable us to behave appropriately? The "why" is fairly obvious: for reasons of survival, the necessary mechanisms to yield perceptual accuracy have evolved. The "how" is more problematic. As good a picture as the eye "takes" of a scene, it falls short of a reproduction of it in several important respects. Chief among these is that the retinal picture is two-dimensional, whereas the world it represents is three-dimensional. Somehow the brain is able to construct a fairly accurate three-dimensional representation of the scene from the two-dimensional retinal image. Although it is true that we perceive depth on the basis of the combined working of our two eyes, merely alluding to such stereoscopic depth by no means solves the problem of how the brain achieves it (see Chapter 5 by T. Poggio). In fact, depth perception by stereopsis is a perfect example of perceptual construction by the brain because we end up with depth perception from two images, neither of which has depth. Furthermore, we achieve depth perception quite well with only one eye. Close an eye in viewing the scene before you; the scene will not noticeably flatten out at all. Therefore, the brain is capable of constructing a three-dimensional scene from information contained within a single two-dimensional image. Nonetheless it can hardly be said that the depth we perceive is *in* the picture the eye receives (see Chapter 8 by V. S. Ramachandran).

The problem of the brain's accurate perceptual construction of the world goes beyond the problem of depth. When we view a circle at a slant from any position other than straight on, for example, it projects an elliptical rather than a circular image to the eye, as is demonstrated by the plate with fruit and the slices of cucumber in the still life photograph (Figure 3.1) in Chapter 3 by E. H. Land. Yet we ordinarily see a circle, not an ellipse. Despite great variability in the particular shape of the retinal image as we move from one position to another, and despite lack of correspondence between that image and the actual shape of the object, our perception remains remarkably stable and accurate. Investigators refer to the stability and accuracy of perception as *constancy*, in this case constancy of shape.

They refer to the correspondence between the percept, or construction, and the external object as *veridicality*, which means truthfulness. Perception is remarkably veridical, although, as we shall see, not perfectly or always so.

Constancy

Constancy is the general rule about perception, not the exception. For example, in viewing the same object from varying distances, we receive images that vary in retinal size, yet they remain much the same size in our perception (see Figure I.2). This size constancy, as many studies show, is perceptual and not simply an act of judgment or knowledge. In other words, objects actually *appear* to be the same size at varying distances. Even animals and infants behave as if their perception of object size, despite variation of distance, is constant; it is unlikely that they would do so if constancy were a matter of reasoning rather than of perception.

Perceptual constancy is also evident when we change our position or orientation in relation to an object. Consider what happens when you tilt your head when looking at an object: the scene hardly looks tilted. This is an example of orientation con-

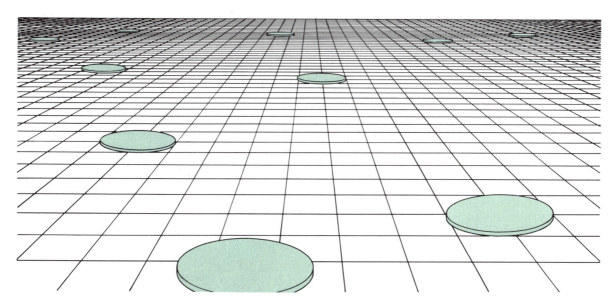

Figure I.2 SIZE CONSTANCY. The equal-sized disks, although producing diminishing retinal images with distance, tend to look equal in size in viewing actual scenes.

(Adapted from "The Processes of Vision," by Ulric Neisser. Copyright © 1968 by SCIENTIFIC AMERICAN. All rights reserved.)

stancy (see Chapter 7 by this author). Or suppose you are moving through space or just turn your head or just move your eyes. The image of the scene sweeps over the retina, but the scene hardly appears to move (position or direction constancy). You are aware that *you* did the moving.

Another type of constancy is of lightness and color. In everyday life, there is continuous change in illumination, whether natural (as by time of day or weather) or artificial (as by the source of light indoors). The result is great change in both the intensity and distribution of spectral light to the eye. Yet, as is evident from the image on the cover, white surfaces don't look darker or black in dim light; by the same token, black ones don't look lighter or white in bright light and red surfaces don't look very different even when seen in the yellow-tinged light of an incandescent bulb. Why surfaces do not appear to vary in lightness or color under such varying conditions of illumination has been another challenging problem to investigators of perception (see Chapter 3 by E. H. Land and Chapter 4 by A. L. Gilchrist).

How does the brain achieve constancy? There are two major schools of thought on this question. One explanation is that the brain engages in an unconscious process akin to reasoning—unconscious inference, the great 19th century scientist Hermann von Helmholtz called it. For example, in the case of size, we can see the distance of the object whose size we are assessing. Therefore, even if the retinal image of the object is small, we perceive the object to be far away, triggering our brain to "compute" that the object is nonetheless large. It is as if we multiply the size of the image (or visual angle, as it is called) by perceived or registered distance. In short, the brain takes account of distance in computing size, of slant in computing shape and of body orientation in computing orientation.

The other explanation is that constancy is given directly by certain kinds of information contained within the retinal image. This view has its roots in the ideas of Ewald Hering, a contemporary of Helmholtz, and in certain of the ideas of the Gestalt psychologists. More recently, it was championed by the late James J. Gibson of Cornell University, perhaps the major figure in the field of perception over the last half century. The explanation of lightness constancy provides a good example of this line of thinking. When the illumination changes, not only does a white, gray or black surface reflect more or less light to the retina, the surface surrounding the

one in question also will receive that altered illumination and also reflect more or less light to the eye. Hering speculated that the neural activity in a region surrounding another region alters the neural activity in the surrounded region. The Gestalt psychologists emphasized *relationships* between stimuli, and one researcher trained in this tradition, Hans Wallach, went on to show in an elegant experiment that if the ratio of light intensity in region A (for example, a disk) to that in region B (for example, a ring around the disk) remains the same, the perceived lightness of the disk will remain unchanged. We might conclude that it is the ratio of light intensity that governs the perceived lightness of surfaces. Because it usually is not affected by changes in illumination—although the absolute intensity *is*—this ratio would explain lightness constancy. As is discussed in Chapter 4, the matter is not quite this simple, but it does seem to be true that there is more information in the stimulus than has previously been thought to be the case.

Illusions and Veridical Perception

I hope that by now the reader can appreciate why the analogy of eye to camera hardly begins to explain our remarkably constant and veridical perception of the world around us. However I hasten to add an important caveat: perception is not always veridical; it is sometimes illusory. Figure I.3 is but one of countless examples. If perception results from lawful constructive processes in the brain, whatever these processes are, is it reasonable to suppose that they never fail to bring a veridical outcome? Failures could occur for many reasons. For example, if the cells in the retina have become fatigued, they won't respond normally to a new stimulus and would alter the neural signals from the retina that are transmitted to the brain (see Chapter 2 by O. E. Favreau and M. C. Corballis). Or suppose the information concerning the slant or depth of an object is prevented from reaching the eye. If we can't see that a circle that is slanted away from us *is* slanted, we may fail to perceive it as a circle and instead misperceive it as an ellipse. Or, conversely, consider how an object that is flat, such as a *drawing* of converging railway tracks, suggests depth to the viewer even though there is no actual depth in the drawing (see Chapter 11 by B. Gillam). In this case, we would expect the constructive process to lead to an illusion. In fact, investigators of perception study illusions because they believe that these may pro-

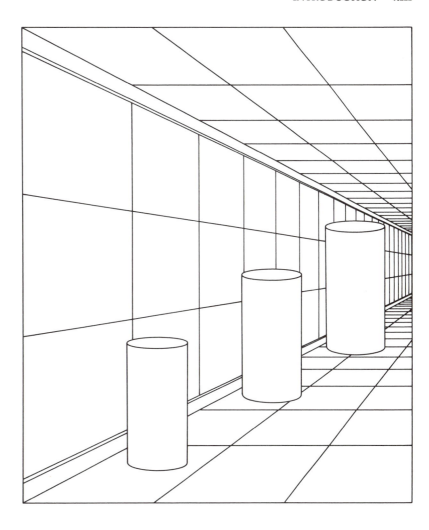

Figure I.3 AN ILLUSION OF SIZE. The three cylinders are equal in size in the picture but look quite unequal. (Adapted from *The Perception of the Visual World* by J. J. Gibson, Houghton Mifflin, Copyright © 1950.)

vide insights into the working of the mind under more ordinary circumstances.

Illusions occur surprisingly often in daily life and are not restricted to the geometrical kind discussed in Chapter 11. For example, in viewing movies or television we perceive motion, yet what we are actually viewing is a succession of stationary pictures. (Chapter 9 by V. S. Ramachandran and S. M. Anstis describes several new insights into how the mind achieves such apparent motion.) Illusions of motion often occur when a large or surrounding object moves near a smaller or surrounded one. For example, the moon appears to move when clouds drift slowly in front of it, an effect referred to as induced motion. Even one's own body can undergo induced motion such as when a nearby train or car moves

slowly and we misperceive ourselves and our own stationary train or car as moving. These illusions of induced motion seem to be a result of stimulus relationships and what the Gestalt psychologists call a "frame of reference."

Perceptual Organization

There is yet another reason why we cannot explain perception simply on the basis of the "picture" that the eye receives. The retinal image is not a picture any more than a photograph is a picture unless there is a viewer to construct it as one. A photograph is nothing more than an arrangement of points reflecting differing intensities and wavelengths. When we view it, however, we group certain points together—for example, all the dark regions near one another within a rectangular region—and we do not group these points with higher-intensity points that surround that region. As a result, we perceive a rectangular shape on a homogeneous background (which we may then go on to recognize as the shape of a book). In short, to perceive the rectangle in the picture, we engage in grouping or organization.

Precisely the same is true about the retinal image. Were we to place a sheet of paper in front of the retina, allowing the picture that the eye-as-camera projects on it to become visible, we would have a kind of photograph, but one as yet unorganized by a mind. If we take away the paper in our thought experiment and allow the light to fall on the millions of separate light-sensitive cells of the retina, we have not changed anything in the logic of the analysis.

Only through the brain's organization of the stimulus pattern of light falling upon the retina can we achieve the perception—a world of separate, shaped, segregated objects. We owe this understanding to early 20th century Gestalt psychologists, who not only pointed out the problem, but

also suggested an answer to it. The organization of the field into distinct, segregated objects, they argued, was based on a set of laws for grouping all the components of the stimulus falling upon the eye (or ear or skin, for that matter). Some of these laws are illustrated in Figure I.4

The concept of grouping or organization helps clarify another important reason for thinking of perception as the end result of a process of construction in the brain. The retinal image, or proximal stimulus, as perception investigators sometimes call it, is ambiguous. Suppose, for example, that some degree of organization has occurred, so that we perceive the objects depicted in Figure I.5. Each is a reversible figure and can be seen in more than one way. Since the stimulus does not change, the change in perception must be brought about by some constructive or reconstructive process in the brain. Various other examples of reversal will be encountered in Chapters 7, 8, 9 and 10.

Another kind of ambiguity about the proximal stimulus is implicit in our earlier discussion of constancy. There we saw that many variations of a stimulus could give rise to the same perception: ellipses of various shapes, as well as circles, can be

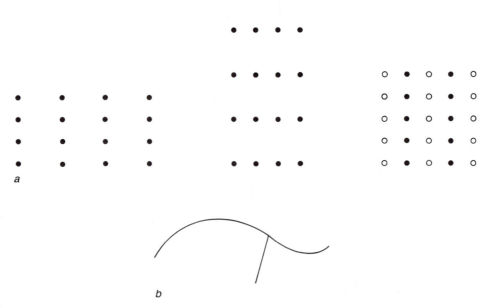

Figure I.4 GESTALT LAWS OF GROUPING. (a) We tend to group the dots in the pattern on the left into columns and those in the middle into rows because of their relative nearness to one another (the law of proximity). In the pattern on the right, we tend to group together the spots that are similar to one another—that is, black dots and white dots—by the law of similarity. In this pattern, the separations between rows are the same as those between columns, which neutralizes the law of proximity. (b) In this pattern we tend to group together the parts of the curved line, excluding the straight line (the law of good continuation).

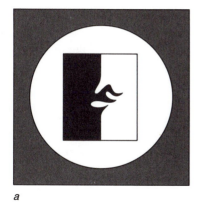
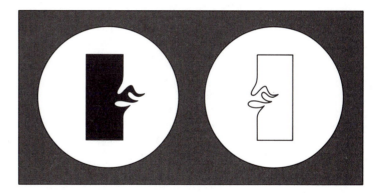

a

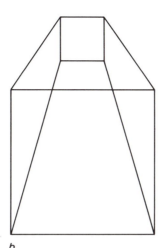

b

Figure I.5 REVERSIBLE PATTERNS. (*a*) A reversible figure-ground pattern shown on the left can be perceived in either one of the two ways shown on the right. (From *An Introduction to Perception* by Irvin Rock. Copyright © 1975 by Irvin Rock. Published by Macmillan.) (*b*) This reversible perspective pattern can be seen either as a box (or hallway) or as a truncated pyramid. A better known example of a perspective reversal pattern, the Necker cube, is shown in Figure 9.6.

perceived as circular shapes in the world, and stimuli of varying retinal sizes can all give rise to the same perception of an object of a particular size. The converse is also true: a retinal image of constant shape or size can produce a variety of differing perceptions. In fact the circumscribed image of an object of any given shape, size, luminance, wavelength or orientation is inherently ambiguous. More information is required before a definite perception will occur.

The necessity for perceptual organization and the reconstruction that occurs in reversing ambiguous figures points up the active role of the brain in perception. So too does the effect of attention. By merely shifting our attention from one object or region to another, we can affect what we perceive. Experiments have confirmed the kind of effect we often experience at a cocktail party, when we can voluntary choose which conversation to listen to and the other conversations essentially are no longer perceived or, if perceived, are perceived only with considerable loss of organization and comprehension. Yet, as noted earlier, segregation of the scene on the basis of the detection of similarities and differences among elements with respect to a single property, such as color, can occur in parallel and therefore, presumably, preattentively (see Chapter 6 by A. Treisman).

Perception and the Brain

So far, I have spoken of constructive processes of *the brain* as the fundamental causes of our perceptions. Few psychologists would disagree with this claim. Yet many investigators often do *not* immediately seek brain-process explanations of perceptual phenomena. Perhaps the main reason is that we first must arrive at reasonable hypotheses of *what kind of process* must be going on. Such hypotheses can then be tested by psychological — or, as we usually say in perception, psychophysical — experimentation. Once we have discovered the functional basis of a perceptual phenomenon, we can begin to investigate the brain mechanism underlying it. Only then do we know what kind of mechanism to look for. A second reason for postponing attempts at brain-mechanism explanations of perceptual effects is that we still know very little about the brain, too little to cope with the complexities of the phenomenon of perception, about which we often know much more.

Therefore, many of the investigators whose chapters appear in this Reader steer clear of speculating about neurophysiological explanations of the phenomena they discuss, not because they do not believe in such explanations, but because they think they are premature. Consider the example of subjective contours discussed in Chapter 10 by G. Kanizsa. The region or figure that acquires these "contours" appears to be even whiter than the surrounding white page (see Figure 10.1, left). Since black segments are used to produce these illusory figures, what could be more plausible than to assume that the whiter-than-white perception is caused by contrast? Contrast is a well-known effect in sensation and perception and is thought to be based on a known neural mechanism called lateral inhibition. If lateral inhibition brings about this lightness effect, it ipso facto explains the subjective contour: the inner white regions would have to seem to have contours if they are lighter than the surrounding white. Yet as the author shows by other examples, this explanation may be incorrect. Subjective contours occur when such contrast cannot be the explanation and they fail to occur when they ought to if contrast were the explanation.

The research described in Chapter 2, however, is an interesting example of the productive mixture of knowledge of facts about perception and of discoveries about neural mechanisms. This may well be because most of the perceptual effects they discuss are of a less complex, sensory kind. For example, we can explain a negative afterimage on the basis of the fatiguing of certain cells in the retina and possibly also explain a negative aftereffect — for example, the apparent tilt of a vertical line — following the inspection of tilted lines on the basis of the fatiguing of the kind of cortical orientation-detector cell discovered by D. H. Hubel and T. N. Wiesel, as described in Chapter 1.

Explaining a phenomenon at a lower (and presumably deeper) level has become a model of scientific progress, for example, explaining the behavior of solids, liquids and gasses by the behavior of molecules. A brain-event explanation of a psychological fact presumably would be an example of such a deeper level explanation. However, some psychologists voice concern that neural explanations may not do justice to important qualities of mental phenomena. My own view is that this concern is unnecessary, because if and when we succeed in arriving at neurophysiological accounts of perceptual effects, we will still need functional explanations to accompany them. Without including them, neural explanations will be unintelligible. A physicist might be able to explain the action of a carburetor at the molecular or even submolecular level, but unless we know what a carburetor *does* in relation to an automobile engine, the explanation won't make any sense.

Perception and Experience

Little has been said so far about the role of past experience and memory in perception. To be sure, if we are talking about recognizing and identifying objects, past experience carried over in memory must be responsible. But what about the role of memory in other perceptual properties and effects, such as those we have been discussing?

Consider first the fact that the eye only provides clear vision in its center, the fovea. The fovea represents a very small part of the visual scene at any moment, roughly the size of a nickel held at arm's length. Yet we do not have the impression that the scene we look at is blurry or that we can only see a tiny portion of it. The reason is that our eyes are in constant motion, moving on the average about four times a second. If we cannot perceive the entire scene clearly on the basis of any single "picture" the retina receives from a stationary eye, but nevertheless can and do easily see the scene as we look at it, then the brain must be integrating these several still "shots" into one coherent structure. To do that, the brain must somehow "know" that the stimulus on the fovea at one moment is located in a certain position in the scene with respect to the stimulus on the fovea at another moment, after one or more eye movements. In short, the perceived object or scene indeed seems to be the result of a process of construction over time.

If we must integrate several foveal views of a scene in order to perceive it in its entirety, memory of some kind must enter into the process. It has been shown that there is indeed a very brief memory of a stimulus on the retina that lasts about a quarter of a second. It is referred to as iconic storage and is more or less an exact representation of the image. So iconic memory may play a role in the overall perception of the scene before us.

What about the effect of longer-range memory on perception? The relative contributions of innately determined, wired-in mechanisms and past experience on perception has been a controversial topic for many centuries. We now know that both factors govern perception. The intricate neural mechanisms the brain uses to pick up information from the retina, which are described in Chapter 1, are surely genetically determined (although, interestingly, if a newborn kitten is deprived of a visual environment containing edges in all orientations, these mechanisms will not mature normally). Moreover, the results of new studies of infant vision indicate that within the first few months of life, infants are able to perceive depth, shape and other properties of objects and even are able to achieve perceptual constancy.

On the other hand, we also know that past experience can affect perception. However, it is important to make a distinction here: what we consciously *know* about a particular stimulus pattern confronting us usually does *not* affect what we perceive. This is close to being a fundamental rule about perception. Perception is more or less autonomous with respect to certain cognitive functions, such as conceptual knowledge and thinking. Illusions, for example, do not disappear merely because we know that they are illusions (see Chapters 2, 9, 10 and 11). Still, past experience, operating below the level of

conscious awareness, in the form of stored memories, *can* affect perception. Consider subjective contours such as those displayed in Chapter 10. Usually they occur when a pattern can be interpreted as one object covering over others that otherwise would be incomplete. It is at least plausible to believe that our past experience has led us to interpret certain patterns as incomplete because of our familiarity with what they look like when they are complete. Past experience certainly also enters into what we perceive when we read, leading us often to misperceive words based on our lexical and semantic knowledge base.

Although I said that perception should be considered separate from other modes of cognition, it does seem to be similar to dreaming and imagery. When we dream, we do see a picture in our mind's eye. From the standpoint of subjective experience alone, it would be difficult to maintain that most dreams are not visual representations of outer objects and events. However, perception is properly defined as the achievement of such mental representations, from the stimulation of a sense organ. By this definition dreams are not perceptions. Since the end product in a dream is so similar to a percept, however, it seems reasonable to suppose that certain similar events must be occurring within the brain, although not in the sense organs, and that these result in the same kind of subjective experience of outer things and happenings. Therefore, the dividing line between perceiving and dreaming may be less sharp than is sometimes thought.

What about imagery? Many people claim that their image of a scene is very similar to their perception of a scene. (I am not referring here to eidetikers, those few individuals who seem to have such a vivid mental picture, or eidetic image, of a scene that they can inspect it and answer specific questions, such as how many windows a house has.) As noted earlier, psychologists have recently become very interested in the relationship between perception and imagery.

A useful overall way of looking at the field of perception is to view it as lying midway on a continuum, with the field of sensory processes at one end and cognition at the other. Investigators of sensory processes are concerned with the physiological mechanisms that mediate our experiences of sensations such as of color, taste and pitch and in which the representation of object structures is not relevant. Investigators of cognition are concerned with principles that account for imagery, learning, memory and thinking. Investigators of perception are concerned with our apprehension of external objects and events. Of course there are no sharp divisions between these overlapping areas of study.

In this introduction, I have tried to explain why there is such a field as perception. The articles selected for this volume present the kinds of problems investigators try to unravel and the methods and approaches they employ. Other investigators are currently at work attempting to fill in the gaps in our understanding of sensory and cognitive processes. Collectively, advances in all of these areas are increasing our knowledge of mind and brain.

Irvin Rock

The Perceptual World

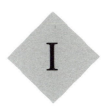

BRAIN MECHANISMS

. . .

Brain Mechanisms of Vision

A functional architecture that may underlie processing of sensory information in the cortex is revealed by studies of the activity and the organization in space of neurons in the primary visual cortex.

• • •

David H. Hubel and Torsten N. Wiesel
September, 1979

Viewed as a kind of invention by evolution, the cerebral cortex must be one of the great success stories in the history of living things. In vertebrates lower than mammals the cerebral cortex is minuscule, if it can be said to exist at all. Suddenly impressive in the lowest mammals, it begins to dominate the brain in carnivores, and it increases explosively in primates; in man it almost completely envelops the rest of the brain, tending to obscure the other parts. The degree to which an animal depends on an organ is an index of the organ's importance that is even more convincing than size, and dependence on the cortex has increased rapidly as mammals have evolved. A mouse without a cortex appears fairly normal, at least to casual inspection; a man without a cortex is almost a vegetable, speechless, sightless, senseless.

Understanding of this large and indispensable organ is still woefully deficient. This is partly because it is very complex, not only structurally but also in its functions, and partly because neurobiologists' intuitions about the functions have so often been wrong. The outlook is changing, however, as techniques improve and as investigators learn how to deal with the huge numbers of intricately connected neurons that are the basic elements of the cortex, with the impulses they carry and with the synapses that connect them. In this chapter we hope to sketch the present state of knowledge of one subdivision of the cortex: the primary visual cortex (also known as the striate cortex or area 17), the most elementary of the cortical regions concerned with vision. That will necessarily lead us into the related subject of visual perception, since the workings of an organ cannot easily be separated from its biological purpose (see Figure 1.1).

The cerebral cortex, a highly folded plate of neural tissue about two millimeters thick, is an outermost crust wrapped over the top of, and to some extent tucked under, the cerebral hemispheres (see Figure 1.2). In man its total area, if it were spread out, would be about 1.5 square feet. (In a 1963 article in SCIENTIFIC AMERICAN one of us gave the area as 20 square feet and was quickly corrected by a neuroanatomist friend in Toronto, who said he thought it was 1.5 square feet—"at least that is what Canadians have.") The folding is presumably mainly the result of such an unlikely structure's having to be packed into a box the size of the skull.

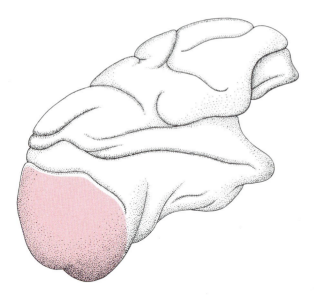 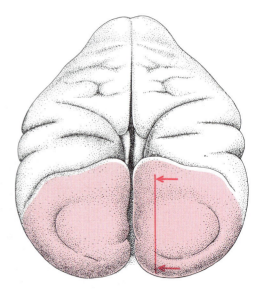

Figure 1.1 PRIMARY VISUAL CORTEX, also known as the striate cortex or area 17, is a region of the cerebral cortex: a layered plate of neurons that envelops the primate brain. In the macaque brain, seen here from the side (*left*) and from above and behind (*right*), the primary visual cortex (*colored areas*) occupies most of the exposed surface of the two occipital lobes. It also curves around the medial surface between the two cerebral hemispheres. It continues in a complex fold underneath the convex outer surface, as is shown in a parasagittal section in Figure 1.2 that was cut along the colored line and is viewed in the direction indicated by the arrows.

A casual glance at cortical tissue under a microscope shows vast numbers of neurons: about 10^5 (100,000) for each square millimeter of surface, suggesting that the cortex as a whole has some 10^{10} (10 billion) neurons. The cell bodies are arranged in half a dozen layers that are alternately cell-sparse and cell-rich. In contrast to these marked changes in cell density in successive layers at different depths in the cortex there is marked uniformity from place to place in the plane of any given layer and in any direction within that plane. The cortex is morphologically rather uniform in two of its dimensions (see Figure 1.3).

One of the first great insights about cortical organization came late in the 19th century, when it was gradually realized that this rather uniform plate of tissue is subdivided into a number of different regions that have very different functions. The evidence came from clinical, physiological and anatomical sources. It was noted that a brain injury, depending on its location, could cause paralysis or blindness or numbness or speech loss; the blindness could be total or limited to half or less of the visual world, and the numbness could involve one limb or a few fingers. The consistency of the relation between a given defect and the location of the lesion gradually led to a charting of the most obvious of these specialized regions, the visual, auditory, somatic sensory (body sensation), speech and motor regions.

In many cases a close look with a microscope at cortex stained for cell bodies showed that in spite of the relative uniformity there were structural variations, particularly in the layering pattern, that correlated well with the clinically defined subdivisions. Additional confirmation came from observations of the location (at the surface of the brain) of the electrical brain waves produced when an animal was stimulated by touching the body, sounding clicks or tones in the ear or flashing light in the eye. Similarly, motor areas could be mapped by stimulating the cortex electrically and noting what part of the animal's body moved.

This systematic mapping of the cortex soon led to a fundamental realization: most of the sensory and motor areas contained systematic two-dimensional maps of the world they represented. Destroying a particular small region of cortex could lead to paralysis of one arm; a similar lesion in another

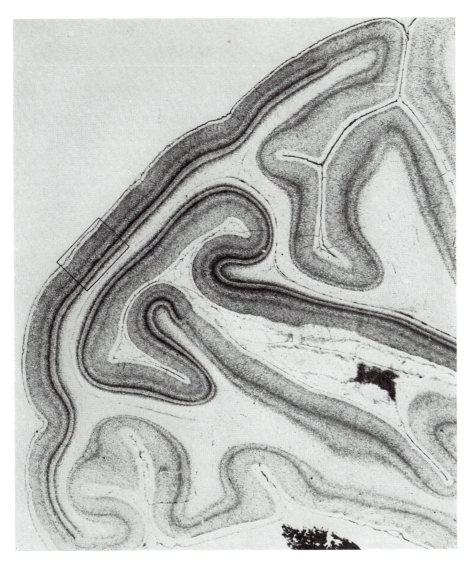

Figure 1.2 SECTION OF VISUAL CORTEX along the colored line in Figure 1.1 was stained by the Nissl method, which makes cell bodies but not fibers visible. The visual cortex is seen to be a continuous layered sheet of neurons about two millimeters thick. The black rectangle outlines a section like the one that is further enlarged in Figure 1.3.

small region led to numbness of one hand or of the upper lip, or blindness in one small part of the visual world; if electrodes were placed on an animal's cortex, touching one limb produced a correspondingly localized series of electric potentials. Clearly the body was systematically mapped onto the somatic sensory and motor areas; the visual world was mapped onto the primary visual cortex, an area on the occipital lobe that in man and in the macaque monkey (the animal in which our investigations have mainly been conducted) covers about 15 square centimeters.

In the primary visual cortex the map is uncomplicated by breaks and discontinuities except for the remarkable split of the visual world down the exact middle, with the left half projected to the right cerebral cortex and the right half projected to the left cortex. The map of the body is more complicated

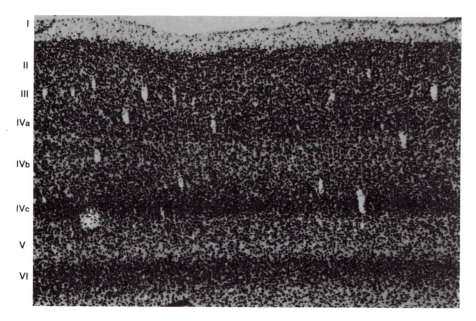

Figure 1.3 CROSS SECTION OF PRIMARY VISUAL CORTEX in the macaque, stained here by the Nissl method and enlarged about 35 diameters, shows the layered struc- **ture and gives the conventional designations of the six layers (*left*). The white gaps are sectioned blood vessels.**

and is still perhaps not completely understood. It is nonetheless systematic, and it is similarly crossed, with the right side of the body projecting to the left hemisphere and the left side projecting to the right hemisphere. (It is worth remarking that no one has the remotest idea why there should be this amazing tendency for nervous-system pathways to cross.)

An important feature of cortical maps is their distortion. The scale of the maps varies as it does in a Mercator projection, the rule for the cortex being that the regions of highest discrimination or delicacy of function occupy relatively more cortical area. For the body surface, a millimeter of surface on the fingers, the lips or the tongue projects to more cortex than a millimeter of trunk, buttocks or back; in vision the central part of the retina has a representation some 35 times more detailed than the far peripheral part.

Important as the advances in mapping cortical projections were, they tended for some time to divert thought from the real problem of just how the brain analyzes information. It was as though the representation could be an end in itself instead of serving a more subtle purpose—as though what the

cortex did was to cater to some little green man who sat inside the head and surveyed images playing across the cortex. In the course of this chapter we shall show that, for vision at least, the world is represented in a far more distorted way; any little green man trying to glean information from the cortical projection would be puzzled indeed.

The first major insight into cortical organization was nonetheless the recognition of this subdivision into areas having widely different functions, with a tendency to ordered mapping. Just how many such areas there are has been a subject of wide speculation. Anatomists' estimates have on the whole been rather high—up to several hundred areas, depending on the individual worker's sensitivity to fine differences in microscopic patterns and sometimes also on his ability to fool himself. Physiologists began with lower estimates, but lately, with more powerful mapping methods, they have been revising their estimates upward. The important basic notion is that information on any given modality such as sight or sound is transmitted first to a primary cortical area and from there, either directly or via the thalamus, to successions of higher areas. A modern guess as to the number of cortical areas might be between 50 and 100.

The second major insight into cortical organization came from the work of the anatomist Santiago Ramón y Cajal and his pupil Rafael Lorente de Nó. This was the realization that the operations the cortex performs on the information it receives are local. What that means can best be understood by considering the wiring diagram that emerged from the Golgi method used by Cajal and Lorente de Nó. In essence the wiring is simple. Sets of fibers bring information to the cortex; by the time several synapses have been traversed the influence of the input has spread vertically to all cell layers; finally several other sets of fibers carry modified messages out of the area. The detailed connections between inputs and outputs differ from one area to the next, but within a given area they seem to be rather stereotyped. What is common to all regions is the local nature of the wiring. The information carried into the cortex by a single fiber can in principle make itself felt through the entire thickness in about three or four synapses, whereas the lateral spread, produced by branching trees of axons and dendrites, is limited for all practical purposes to a few millimeters, a small proportion of the vast extent of the cortex.

The implications of this are far-reaching. Whatever any given region of the cortex does, it does locally. At stages where there is any kind of detailed, systematic topographical mapping the analysis must be piecemeal. For example, in the somatic sensory cortex the messages concerning one finger can be combined and compared with an input from elsewhere on that same finger or with input from a neighboring finger, but they can hardly be combined with the influence from the trunk or from a foot. The same applies to the visual world. Given the detailed order of the input to the primary visual cortex, there is no likelihood that the region will do anything to correlate information coming in from both far above and far below the horizon, or from both the left and the right part of the visual scene. It follows that this cannot by any stretch of the imagination be the place where actual perception is enshrined. Whatever these cortical areas are doing, it must be some kind of local analysis of the sensory world. One can only assume that as the information on vision or touch or sound is relayed from one

cortical area to the next, the map becomes progressively more blurred and the information carried more abstract.

Even though the Golgi-method studies of the early 1900's made it clear that the cortex must perform local analyses, it was half a century before physiologists had the least inkling of just what the analysis was in any area of the cortex. The first understanding came in the primary visual area, which is now the best-understood of any cortical region and is still the only one where the analysis and consequent transformations of information are known in any detail. After describing the main transformations that take place in the primary visual cortex we shall go on to show how increasing understanding of these cortical functions has revealed an entire world of architectural order that is otherwise inaccessible to observation.

We can best begin by tracing the visual path in a primate from the retina to the cortex (see Figure 1.4). The output from each eye is conveyed to the brain by about a million nerve fibers bundled together in the optic nerve. These fibers are the axons of the ganglion cells of the retina. The messages from the light-sensitive elements, the rods and cones, have already traversed from two to four synapses and have involved four other types of retinal cells before they arrive at the ganglion cells, and a certain amount of sophisticated analysis of the information has already taken place.

A large fraction of the optic-nerve fibers pass uninterrupted to two nests of cells deep in the brain called the lateral geniculate nuclei, where they make synapses. The lateral geniculate cells in turn send their axons directly to the primary visual cortex. From there, after several synapses, the messages are sent to a number of further destinations: neighboring cortical areas and also several targets deep in the brain. One contingent even projects back to the lateral geniculate bodies; the function of this feedback path is not known. The main point for the moment is that the primary visual cortex is in no sense the end of the visual path. It is just one stage, probably an early one in terms of the degree of abstraction of the information it handles.

As a result of the partial crossing of the optic nerves in the optic chiasm, the geniculate and the cortex on the left side are connected to the two left

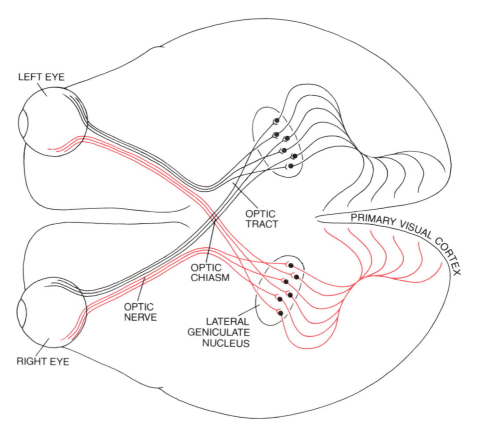

Figure 1.4 VISUAL PATHWAY is traced schematically in the human brain, seen here from below. The output from the retina is conveyed, by ganglion-cell axons bundled in the optic nerves, to the lateral geniculate nuclei; about half of the axons cross over to the opposite side of the brain, so that a representation of each half of the visual scene is projected on the geniculate of the opposite hemisphere. Neurons in the geniculates send their axons to the primary visual cortex.

half retinas and are therefore concerned with the right half of the visual scene, and the converse is the case for the right geniculate and the right cortex. Each geniculate and each cortex receives input from both eyes, and each is concerned with the opposite half of the visual world, as shown in Figure 1.4.

To examine the workings of this visual pathway our strategy since the late 1950's has been (in principle) simple. Beginning, say, with the fibers of the optic nerve, we record with microelectrodes from a single nerve fiber and try to find out how we can most effectively influence the firing by stimulating the retina with light. For this one can use patterns of light of every conceivable size, shape and color, bright on a dark background or the reverse, and stationary or moving. It may take a long time, but

sooner or later we satisfy ourselves that we have found the best stimulus for the cell being tested, in this case a ganglion cell of the retina. (Sometimes we are wrong!) We note the results and then go on to another fiber. After studying a few hundred cells we may find that new types become rare. Satisfied that we know roughly how the neurons at this stage work, we proceed to the next stage (in this case the geniculate) and repeat the process. Comparison of the two sets of results can tell us something about what the geniculate does. We then go on to the next stage, the primary cortex, and repeat the procedure.

Working in this way, one finds that both a retinal ganglion cell and a geniculate cell respond best to a roughly circular spot of light of a particular size in a particular part of the visual field. The size is critical because each cell's receptive field (the patch of retinal receptor cells supplying the cell) is divided, with an excitatory center and an inhibitory surround (an ON-center cell) or exactly the reverse configuration (an OFF-center cell). This is the center-surround configuration first described by Stephen W. Kuffler at the Johns Hopkins University School of Medicine in 1953. A spot exactly filling the center of an ON-center cell is therefore a more effective stimulus than a larger spot that invades the inhibitory area, or than diffuse light. A line stimulus (a bar of light) is effective if it covers a large part of the center region and only a small part of the surround. Because these cells have circular symmetry they respond well to such a line stimulus whatever its orientation. To sum up, the retinal ganglion cells and the cells of the lateral geniculate—the cells supplying the input to the visual cortex—are cells with concentric, center-surround receptive fields. They are primarily concerned not with assessing levels of illumination but rather with making a comparison between the light level in one small area of the visual scene and the average illumination of the immediate surround (see Figures 1.5 and 1.6a).

T he first of the two major transformations accomplished by the visual cortex is the re-

arrangement of incoming information so that most of its cells respond not to spots of light but to specifically oriented line segments. There is a wide variety of cell types in the cortex, some simpler and some more complex in their response properties, and one soon gains an impression of a kind of hierarchy, with simpler cells feeding more complex ones. In the monkey there is first of all a large group of cells that behave (as far as is known) just like geniculate cells: they have circularly symmetrical fields. These cells are all in the lower part of one layer, called layer IV, which is precisely the layer that receives the lion's share of the geniculate input. It makes sense that these least sophisticated cortical cells should be the ones most immediately connected to the input.

Cells outside layer IV all respond best to specifically oriented line segments. A typical cell responds only when light falls in a particular part of the visual world, but illuminating that area diffusely has little effect or none, and small spots of light are not much better. The best response is obtained when a line that has just the right tilt is flashed in the region or, in some cells, is swept across the region. The most effective orientation varies from cell to cell and is usually defined sharply enough so that a change of 10 to 20 degrees clockwise or coun-

RIGHT EYE

LEFT EYE

RIGHT EYE

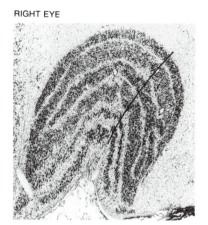
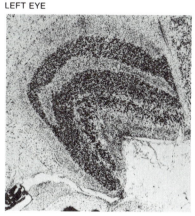
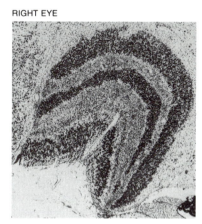

Figure 1.5 LATERAL GENICULATE NUCLEUS of a normal monkey (*left*) is a layered structure in which cells in layers 1, 4 and 6 (*numbered from bottom to top*) receive their input from the eye on the opposite side and those in layers 2, 3 and 5 receive information from the eye on the same side. The maps are in register, so that the neurons along any radius (*black line*) receive signals from the same part of the visual scene. The layered nature of the input is demonstrated in the two geniculates of an animal that had vision in the left eye only (*two micrographs at right*): in each geniculate cells in the three layers with input from right eye have atrophied. Geniculates are enlarged 9 diameters.

a *b* *c*

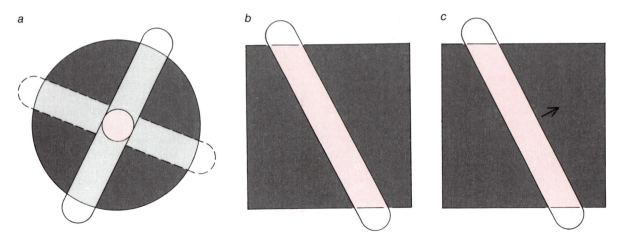

Figure 1.6 RETINAL GANGLION CELLS and neurons in the lateral geniculate nucleus have circular fields with either an excitatory center and an inhibitory surround (*a*) or the opposite arrangement. If it falls on the center, a spot or bar of light stimulates a response from such a cell. The cortical cells that receive signals directly from the geniculate have circularly symmetrical fields; those farther along the pathway respond only to a line stimulus in a particular orientation. A "simple" cell (*b*) responds to such a line stimulus only in a particular part of its field. A "complex" cell (*c*) responds to a precisely oriented line regardless of where it is in its field and also to one moving in a particular direction (*arrow*).

terclockwise reduces the response markedly or abolishes it. (It is hard to convey the precision of this discrimination. If 10 to 20 degrees sounds like a wide range, one should remember that the angle between 12 o'clock and one o'clock is 30 degrees.) A line at 90 degrees to the best orientation almost never evokes any response (see Figure 1.6*b*).

Depending on the particular cell, the stimulus may be a bright line on a dark background or the reverse, or it may be a boundary between light and dark regions. If it is a line, the thickness is likely to be important; increasing it beyond some optimal width reduces the response, just as increasing the diameter of a spot does in the case of ganglion and geniculate cells. Indeed, for a particular part of the visual field the geniculate receptive-field centers and the optimal cortical line widths are comparable.

Neurons with orientation specificity vary in their complexity. The simplest, which we call "simple" cells, behave as though they received their input directly from several cells with center-surround, circularly symmetrical fields—the type of cells found in layer IV. The response properties of these simple cells, which respond to an optimally oriented line in a narrowly defined location, can most easily be accounted for by requiring that the centers of the incoming center-surround fields all be excitatory or all be inhibitory, and that they lie along a straight line. At present we have no direct evidence for this scheme, but it is attractive because of its simplicity and because certain kinds of indirect evidence support it. According to the work of Jennifer S. Lund of the University of Washington School of Medicine, who in the past few years has done more than anyone else to advance the Golgi-stain anatomy of this cortical area, the cells in layer IV project to the layers just above, which is roughly where the simple cells are found.

The second major group of orientation-specific neurons are the far more numerous "complex" cells. They come in a number of subcategories, but their main feature is that they are less particular about the exact position of a line. Complex cells behave as though they received their input from a number of simple cells, all with the same receptive-field orientation but differing slightly in the exact location of their fields. This scheme readily explains the strong steady firing evoked in a complex cell as a line is kept in the optimal orientation and is swept across the receptive field. With the line optimally oriented many cells prefer one direction of movement to the opposite direction. Several possible circuits have been proposed to explain this behavior, but the exact mechanism is still not known (see Figure 1.6c).

Although there is no direct evidence that orientation-sensitive cells have anything to do with visual perception, it is certainly tempting to think they represent some early stage in the brain's analysis of visual forms. It is worth asking which cells at this early stage would be expected to be turned on by some very simple visual form, say a dark blob on a light background. Any cell whose receptive field is entirely inside or outside the boundaries of such an image will be completely unaffected by the figure's presence because cortical cells effectively ignore diffuse changes in the illumination of their entire receptive fields.

The only cells to be affected will be those whose field is cut by the borders. For the circularly symmetrical cells the ones most strongly influenced will be those whose center is grazed by a boundary (because for them the excitatory and inhibitory subdivisions are most unequally illuminated). For the orientation-specific cells the only ones to be activated will be those whose optimal orientation happens to coincide with the prevailing direction of the border. And among these the simple cells will be much more exacting than the complex ones, responding optimally only when the border falls along a line separating an excitatory and an inhibitory region. It is important to realize that this part of the cortex is operating only locally, on bits of the form; how the entire form is analyzed or handled by the brain—how this information is worked on and synthesized at later stages, if indeed it is—is still not known.

The second major function of the monkey visual cortex is to combine the inputs from the two eyes. In the lateral geniculate nuclei a neuron may respond to stimulation of the left eye or of the right one, but no cell responds to stimulation of both eyes. This may seem surprising, since each geniculate receives inputs from both eyes, but the fact is that the geniculates are constructed in a way that keeps inputs from the two eyes segregated. Each geniculate body is divided into six layers, three left-eye layers interdigitated with three right-eye ones. The opposite-side half of the visual world is mapped onto each layer (with the six maps in precise register, so that in a radial pathway traversing

the six layers the receptive fields of all the cells encountered have virtually identical positions in the visual field). Since any one layer has input from only one eye, the individual cells of that layer must be monocular (see Figures 1.4 and 1.5).

Even in the visual cortex the neurons to which the geniculate cells project directly, the circularly symmetrical cells in layer IV, are all (as far as we can tell) strictly monocular; so are all the simple cells. Only at the level of the complex cells do the paths from the two eyes converge, and even there the blending of information is incomplete and takes a special form. About half of the complex cells are monocular, in the sense that any one cell can be activated only by stimulating one eye. The rest of the cells can be influenced independently by both eyes.

If one maps the right-eye and left-eye receptive fields of a binocular cell (by stimulating first through one eye and then through the other) and compares the two fields, the fields turn out to have identical positions, levels of complexity, orientation and directional preference; everything one learns about the cell by stimulating one eye is confirmed through the other eye. There is only one exception: if first one eye and then the other are tested with identical stimuli, the two responses are usually not quantitatively identical; in many cases one eye is dominant, consistently producing a higher frequency of firing than the other eye (see Figure 1.7).

From cell to cell all degrees of ocular dominance can be found, from complete monopoly by one eye through equality to exclusive control by the other eye. In the monkey the cells with a marked eye preference are somewhat commoner than the cells in which the two eyes make about equal contributions. Apparently a binocular cell in the primary visual cortex has connections to the two eyes that are qualitatively virtually identical, but the density of the two sets of connections is not necessarily the same.

It is remarkable enough that the elaborate sets of wiring that produce specificity of orientation and of direction of movement and other special properties should be present in two duplicate copies. It is perhaps even more surprising that all of this can be observed in a newborn animal. The wiring is mostly innate, and it presumably is genetically determined. (In one particular respect, however, some maturation of binocular wiring does take place mostly after birth.)

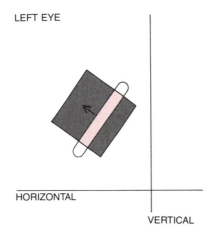

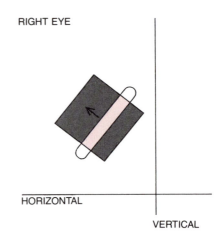

Figure 1.7 BINOCULAR CELL in the cortex can be influenced independently by both eyes or more strongly by both eyes together. Here the left-eye and right-eye fields are mapped for a complex cell whose receptive field is in the upper left quadrant of the visual field. (The lines represent the horizontal and vertical meridians of the field, intersecting at the point of fixation.) The two receptive fields are identical, but the amount of response may differ depending on whether the left eye or the right eye is stimulated. Preference for one eye is called ocular dominance.

We now turn to a consideration of the way these cells are grouped in the cortex. Are cells with similar characteristics—complexity, receptive-field position, orientation and ocular dominance—grouped together or scattered at random? From the description so far it will be obvious that cells of like complexity tend to be grouped in layers, with the circularly symmetrical cells low in layer IV, the simple cells just above them and the complex cells in layers II, III, V and VI. Complex cells can be further subcategorized, and the ones found in each layer are in a number of ways very different.

These differences from layer to layer take on added interest in view of the important discovery, confirmed by several physiologists and anatomists during the past few decades, that fibers projecting from particular layers of the cortex have particular destinations. For example, in the visual cortex the deepest layer, layer VI, projects mainly (perhaps only) back to the lateral geniculate body; layer V projects to the superior colliculus, a visual station in the midbrain; layers II and III send their projections to other parts of the cortex. This relation between layer and projection site probably deserves to be ranked as a third major insight into cortical organization.

The next stimulus variable to be considered is the position of the receptive field in the visual field. In describing the lateral geniculate nucleus we pointed out that in each layer the opposite-half visual field forms an ordered topographical map. In the projection from lateral geniculate to primary visual cortex this order is preserved, producing a cortical map of the visual field. Given this ordered map it is no surprise that neighboring cells in this part of the cortex always have receptive fields that are close together; usually, in fact, they overlap. If one plunges a microelectrode into the cortex at a right angle to the surface and records from cell after cell (as many as 100 or 200 of them) in successively deeper layers, again the receptive fields mostly overlap, with each new field heaped on all the others. The extent of the entire pile of fields is usually several times the size of any one typical field (see Figure 1.8).

There is some variation in the size of these receptive fields. Some of the variation is tied to the layering: the largest fields in any penetration tend to be in layers III, V and VI. The most important variation, however, is linked to eccentricity, or the distance of a cell's receptive field from the center of gaze. The size of the fields and the extent of the associated scatter in the part of the cortex that maps the center of gaze are tiny compared to the size and amount of scatter in the part that maps the far periphery. We call the pile of superimposed fields that are mapped in a penetration beginning at any point on the cortex the "aggregate field" of that

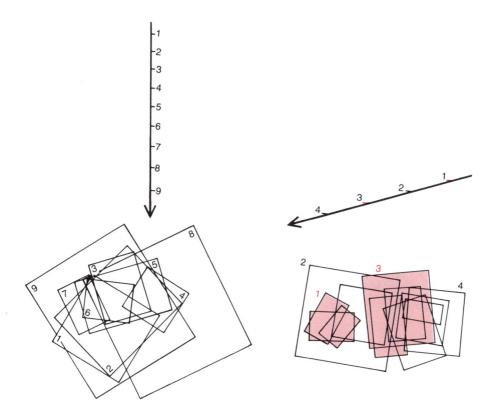

Figure 1.8 POSITIONS OF RECEPTIVE FIELDS (*numbered 1 to 9*) of cortical neurons mapped by an electrode penetrating at roughly a right angle to the surface are essentially the same (*left*), although the fields are different sizes and there is some scatter. In an oblique penetration (*right*) from two to four cells were recorded, at .1-milli-meter intervals, at each of four sites (*numbered from 1 to 4*) one millimeter apart. Each group includes various sizes and some scatter, but now there is also a systematic drift: fields of each successive group of cells are somewhat displaced.

point. The size of the aggregate field is obviously a function of eccentricity.

If the electrode penetrates in an oblique direction, almost parallel to the surface, the scatter in field position from cell to cell is again evident, but now there is superimposed on the scatter a consistent drift in field position, its direction dictated by the topographical map of the visual fields. And an interesting regularity is revealed: it turns out that moving the electrode about one or two millimeters always produces a displacement in visual field that is roughly enough to take one into an entirely new region. The movement in the visual field, in short, is about the same as the size of the aggregate receptive field. For the primary visual cortex this holds wherever the recording is made. At the center of gaze the

fields and their associated scatter are tiny, but so is the displacement corresponding to a one-millimeter movement along the cortex. With increasing eccentricity (farther out in the visual field) both the field and scatter and the displacement become larger, in parallel fashion. It seems that everywhere a block of cortex about one or two millimeters in size is what is needed to take care of a region of the visual world equivalent to the size of an aggregate field.

These observations suggest the way the visual cortex solves a basic problem: how to analyze the visual scene in detail in the central part and much more crudely in the periphery. In the retina, which has the same problem, for obvious optical reasons the number of millimeters corresponding to a degree of visual field is constant. The retina handles the central areas in great detail by having huge numbers of ganglion cells, each subserving a tiny area of central visual field; the layer of ganglion cells in the central part of the retina is thick, whereas in the outlying parts of the retina it is very thin. The cortex, in contrast, seems to want to be uniform in thickness everywhere. Here there are none of the optical constraints imposed on the retina, and so area is simply allotted in amounts corresponding to the problem at hand.

The machinery in any square millimeter of cortex is presumably about the same as in any other. A few thousand geniculate fibers enter such a region, the cortex does its thing and perhaps 50,000 fibers leave—whether a small part of the visual world is represented in great detail or a larger part in correspondingly less detail. The uniformity of the cortex is suggested, as we indicated at the outset, by the appearance of stained sections. It is compellingly confirmed when we examine the architecture further, looking specifically at orientation and at ocular dominance.

For orientation we inquire about groupings of cells just as we did with field position, looking first at two cells sitting side by side. Two such cells almost invariably have the same optimal stimulus orientation. If the electrode is inserted in a direction perpendicular to the surface, all the cells along the path of penetration have identical or almost identical orientations (except for the cells deep in layer IV, which have no optimal orientation at all). In two perpendicular penetrations a millimeter or so apart, however, the two orientations observed are usually different. The cortex must therefore be subdivided by some kind of vertical partitioning into regions of constant receptive-field orientation. When we came on this system almost 20 years ago, it intrigued us because it fitted so well with the hierarchical schemes we had proposed to explain how complex cells are supplied by inputs from simple cells: the circuit diagrams involve connections between cells whose fields cover the same part of the visual world and that respond to the same line orientation. It seemed eminently reasonable that strongly interconnected cells should be grouped together.

If the cortex is diced up into small regions of constant receptive-field orientation, can one say anything more about the three-dimensional shape of the regions than that their walls are perpendicular to the surface? Are neighboring regions related in any systematic way or are regions subserving all the possible orientations scattered over the cortex at random? We began to study these questions simply by penetrating the cortex obliquely or parallel to the surface. When we first did this experiment in about 1961, the result was so surprising that we could hardly believe it. Instead of a random assortment of successive orientations there was an amazing orderliness. Each time the electrode moved forward as little as 25 or 50 micrometers (thousandths of a millimeter) the optimal orientation changed by a small step, about 10 degrees on the average; the steps continued in the same direction, clockwise or counterclockwise, through a total angle of anywhere from 90 to 270 degrees (see Figure 1.9). Occasionally such a sequence would reverse direction suddenly, from a clockwise progression to a counterclockwise one or vice versa. These reversals were unpredictable, usually coming after steady progressions of from 90 to 270 degrees.

Since making this first observation we have seen similar order in almost every monkey. Either there is a steady progression in orientation or, less frequently, there are stretches in which orientation stays constant. The successive changes in orientation are small enough so that it is hard to be sure that the regions of constant orientation are finite in size; it could be that the optimal orientation changes in some sense continuously as the electrode moves along the cortex.

We became increasingly interested in the three-dimensional shape of these regional subdivisions. From considerations of geometry alone the existence of small or zero changes in every direction during a horizontal or tangential penetration points to parallel slabs of tissue containing cells with like orientation specificity, with each slab perpendicular to the surface. The slabs would not necessarily be planar, like slices of bread; seen from above they might well have the form of swirls, which could easily explain the reversals in the direction of orientation changes. Recording large numbers of cells in several parallel electrode penetrations seemed to confirm this prediction, but it was hard to examine more than a tiny region of brain with the microelectrode.

Fortunately an ideal anatomical method was invented at just the right time for us. This was the 2-deoxyglucose technique for assessing brain activity, devised by Louis Sokoloff and his group at the National Institute of Mental Health [see "The Chemistry of the Brain," by Leslie L. Iversen; SCIENTIFIC AMERICAN, September, 1979; Offprint 1441].

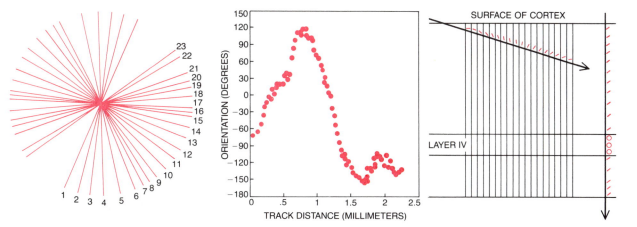

Figure 1.9 ORIENTATION PREFERENCES of 23 neurons encountered as a microelectrode penetrated the cortex obliquely changed steadily in a counterclockwise direction (*left*). A similar experiment (*center*) revealed several reversals in direction. Such results, together with the observation that a microelectrode penetrating the cortex perpendicularly encounters only cells that prefer the same orientation (apart from the circularly symmetrical cells in layer IV with no preferred orientation), suggest that the cortex is subdivided into roughly parallel slabs of tissue, called orientation columns, containing neurons with like orientation specificity (*right*).

The method capitalizes on the fact that brain cells depend mainly on glucose as a source of metabolic energy and that the closely similar compound 2-deoxyglucose can to some extent masquerade as glucose. If deoxyglucose is injected into an animal, it is taken up actively by neurons as though it were glucose; the more active the neuron, the greater the uptake. The compound begins to be metabolized, but for reasons best known to biochemists the sequence stops with a metabolite that cannot cross the cell wall and therefore accumulates within the cell.

The Sokoloff procedure is to inject an animal with deoxyglucose that has been labeled with the radioactive isotope carbon 14, stimulate the animal in a way calculated to activate certain neurons and then immediately examine the brain for radioactivity, which reveals active areas where cells will have taken up more deoxyglucose than those in quiescent areas. The usual way of examining the brain for this purpose is to cut very thin slices of it (as one would for microscopic examination) and press them against a photographic plate sensitive to the radioactive particles. When the film is developed, any areas that were in contact with radioactive material are seen as dark masses of developed silver grains. Together with Michael P. Stryker we adapted the Sokoloff method to our problem, injecting an anesthetized animal with deoxyglucose and then moving a pattern of black and white vertical stripes back and forth 1.5 meters in front of the animal for 45 minutes. We then cut the brain into slices, either perpendicular to the surface of the cortex or parallel to it.

The autoradiographs quickly confirmed the physiological results. Sections cut perpendicular to the surface showed narrow bands of radioactivity about every 570 micrometers (roughly half a millimeter), extending through the full thickness of the cortex. Evidently these were the regions containing cells responsive to vertical lines. The deep part of layer IV was uniformly radioactive, as was expected from the fact that the cells in the layer have circularly symmetrical receptive fields and show no orientation selectivity (see Figure 1.10).

Sections cut parallel to the surface showed an unexpectedly complex set of periodically spaced bands, often swirling, frequently branching and rejoining, only here and there forming regular parallel slabs. What was particularly striking was the uniformity of the distance from one band to the next over the entire cortex. This fitted perfectly with the idea of a uniform cortex. Moreover, the distance between stripes fitted well with the idea that the cortical machinery must repeat itself at least every millimeter. If the distance were, for example, 10 millimeters from vertical through 180 degrees and back to vertical, sizable parts of the visual field

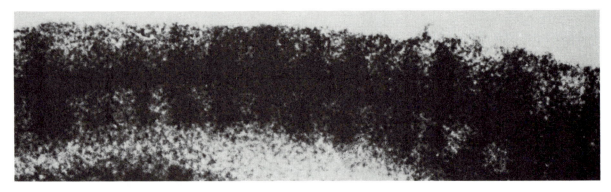

Figure 1.10 ORIENTATION COLUMNS are visualized as anatomical structures in a deoxyglucose autoradiograph made by the authors and Michael P. Stryker. Radioactively labeled deoxyglucose was injected into a monkey; it was taken up primarily by active neurons, and an early metabolite accumulated in the cells. Immediately after the injection the animal was stimulated with a pattern of vertical stripes, so that cells responding to vertical lines were most active and became most radioactive. In this section perpendicular to surface active-cell regions are narrow bands about .5 millimeter apart. Layer IV (with no orientation preference) is, as expected, uniformly radioactive.

would lack cells sensitive to any given orientation, making for a sketchy and extremely bizarre representation of the visual scene (see Figure 1.11).

The final variable whose associated architecture needs to be considered is eye preference. In microelectrode studies neighboring cells proved almost invariably to prefer the same eye. If in vertical penetrations the first cell we encountered preferred the right eye, then so did all the cells, right down to the bottom of layer VI; if the first cell preferred the left eye, so did all the rest. Any penetration favored one eye or the other with equal probability. (Since the cells of layer IV are monocular, there it was a

Figure 1.11 ORIENTATION PATTERN, seen face on, is unexpectedly complex. This deoxyglucose autoradiograph is of a section tangential to the somewhat curved layers of the cortex. The darker regions represent continuously labeled layer IV. In the other layers the orientation regions are intricately curved bands, something like the walls of a maze seen from above, but distance from one band to next is uniform.

matter not of eye preference but of eye monopoly.) If the penetration was oblique or horizontal, there was an alternation of left and right preferences, with a rather abrupt switchover about every half millimeter. The cortex thus proved to be diced up into a second set of regions separated by vertical walls that extend through the full cortical thickness. The ocular-dominance system was apparently quite independent of the orientation system, because in oblique or tangential penetrations the two sequences had no apparent relation to each other (see Figure 1.12).

The basis of these ocular-dominance columns, as they have come to be called, seems to be quite simple. The terminals of geniculate fibers, some subserving the left eye and others the right, group themselves as they enter the cortex so that in layer IV there is no mixing. This produces left-eye and right-eye patches at roughly half-millimeter intervals. A neuron above or below layer IV receives connections from that layer from up to about a millimeter away in every direction. Probably the strongest connections are from the region of layer IV closest to the neuron, so that it is presumably dominated by whichever eye feeds that region.

Again we were most curious to learn what these left-eye and right-eye regions might look like in three dimensions; any of several geometries could

lead to the cross-sectional appearance the physiology had suggested. The answer first came from studies with the silver-degeneration method for mapping connections, devised by Walle J. H. Nauta of the Massachusetts Institute of Technology. Since then we have found three other independent anatomical methods for demonstrating these columns.

A particularly effective method (because it enables one to observe in a single animal the arrangement of columns over the entire primary visual cortex) is based on the phenomenon of axonal transport. The procedure is to inject a radioactively labeled amino acid into an area of nervous tissue. A cell body takes up the amino acid, presumably incorporates it into a protein and then transports it along the axon to its terminals. When we injected the material into one eye of a monkey, the retinal ganglion cells took it up and transported it along their axons, the optic-nerve fibers. We could then examine the destinations of these fibers in the lateral geniculate nuclei by coating tissue slices with a silver emulsion and developing the emulsion; the radioactive label showed up clearly in the three complementary layers of the geniculate on each side.

This method does not ordinarily trace a path from one axon terminal across a synapse to the next neuron and its terminals, however, and we wanted

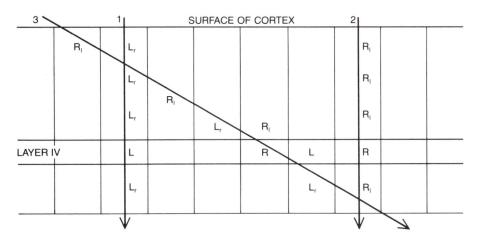

Figure 1.12 OCULAR DOMINANCE was revealed in one typical vertical penetration of the cortex (1), where a microelectrode encounters only cells that respond preferentially to the left eye (L,) and, in layer IV, cells that respond only to the left eye (L). In another vertical penetration (2) the cells all have right-eye dominance (R,) or, in layer IV, are driven exclusively by the right eye (R). An oblique penetration (3) shows regular alternation of dominance. Repeated penetrations suggest subdivisions with a cross-sectional width of about .4 millimeter and with walls perpendicular to the cortical surface and layers: the ocular-dominance columns.

to follow the path all the way to the cortex. In 1971 Bernice Grafstein of the Cornell University Medical College discovered that after a large enough injection in the eye of a mouse some of the radioactive material escaped from the optic-nerve terminals and was taken up by the cells in the geniculate and transported along their axons to the cortex. We had the thought that a similarly large injection in a monkey, combined with autoradiography, might demonstrate the geniculate terminals from one eye in layer IV of the visual cortex.

Our first attempt yielded dismayingly negative results, with only faint hints of a few silver grains visible in layer IV. It was only after several weeks that we realized that by resorting to dark-field microscopy we could take advantage of the light-scattering properties of silver grains and so increase the sensitivity of the method. We borrowed a dark-field condenser, and when we looked at our first slide under the microscope, there shining in all their glory were the periodic patches of label in layer IV (see Figures 1.13 and 1.14).

The next step was to try to see the pattern face on by sectioning the cortex parallel to its surface. The monkey cortex is dome-shaped, and so a section parallel to the surface and tangent to layer IV shows

that layer as a circle or an oval, while a section below layer IV shows it as a ring. By assembling a series of such ovals and rings from a set of sections one can reconstruct the pattern over a wide expanse of cortex.

From the reconstructions it was immediately obvious that the main overall pattern is one of parallel stripes representing terminals belonging to the injected eye, separated by gaps representing the other eye. The striping pattern is not regular like wallpaper. (We remind ourselves occasionally that this is, after all, biology!) Here and there a stripe representing one eye branches into two stripes, or else it ends blindly at a point where a stripe from the other eye branches. The irregularities are commonest near the center of gaze and along the line that maps the horizon. The stripes always seem to be perpendicular to the border between the primary visual cortex and its neighbor, area 18, and here the regularity is greatest. Such general rules seem to apply to all macaque brains, although the details of the pattern vary from one individual to the next and even from one hemisphere to the other in the same monkey (see Figures 1.15 and 1.16).

The width of a set of two stripes is constant, about .8 millimeter, over the entire primary visual cortex, once more emphasizing the uniformity of

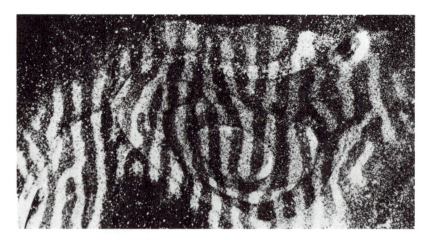

Figure 1.13 ANATOMICAL CONFIRMATION of ocular-dominance columns came from various staining methods and from axonal-transport autoradiographs such as those shown in color in Figures 1.14 and 1.15. This composite autoradiograph visualizing the pattern over an area some 10 millimeters wide was made by cutting out and pasting together the regions representing layer IV in a number of parallel sections, the one in Figure 1.15 and others at different depths.

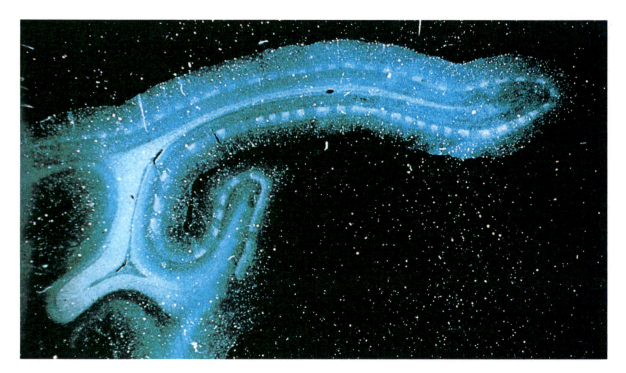

Figure 1.14 OCULAR-DOMINANCE COLUMNS are revealed as periodic bright patches in this autoradiograph of macaque monkey cortex. In these slabs of cortex, seen in cross section in a brain slice cut perpendicularly to the surface, are regions in which all neurons respond more actively to the right eye than to the left; dark regions separating the bright patches are columns of left-eye pref- **erence. A radioactively labeled amino acid injected into the right eye of an anesthetized animal was taken up by cell bodies in the retina and transported via the lateral geniculate nucleus to cells in the cortex. A slice coated with photographic emulsion was exposed for several months and then developed. Exposed silver grains form light-scattering patches that represent the columns.**

the cortex. Again the widths fit perfectly with the idea that all of the apparatus needed to look after an area the size of an aggregate field must be contained within any square millimeter of cortex. The two techniques, deoxyglucose labeling and amino acid transport, have the great advantage of being mutually compatible, so that we have been able to apply both together, one to mark orientation lines and the other to see the ocular-dominance columns. The number of brains examined so far is too small to justify any final conclusions, but the two systems appear to be quite independent, neither parallel nor at right angles but intersecting at random.

The function served by ocular-dominance columns is still a mystery. We know there are neurons with all grades of eye preference throughout the entire binocular part of the visual fields, and it may

be that a regular, patterned system of converging inputs guarantees that the distribution will be uniform, with neither eye favored by accident in any one place. Why there should be all these grades of eye preference everywhere is itself not clear, but our guess is that it has something to do with stereoscopic depth perception.

Given what has been learned about the primary visual cortex, it is clear that one can consider an elementary piece of cortex to be a block about a millimeter square and two millimeters deep. To know the organization of this chunk of tissue is to know the organization for all of area 17; the whole must be mainly an iterated version of this elementary unit (see Figure 1.17). Of course the elementary unit should not be thought of as a discrete, separa-

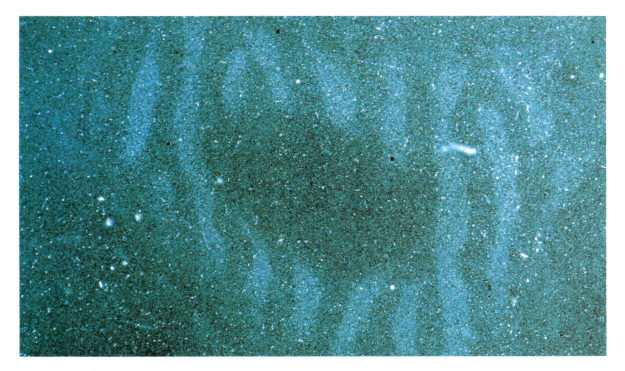

Figure 1.15 DOMINANCE PATTERN is seen face on in an axonal-transport autoradiograph of a brain section parallel to the surface of the primary visual cortex. As can be seen in the autoradiograph in Figure 1.14, the label is brightest in layer IV. This is the level at which the axons bringing visual information to the cortex terminate and where the label therefore accumulates. This section was cut in a plane tangential to the dome-shaped surface of the cortex and just below layer IV, which therefore appears as a ring of roughly parallel bright bands. These are the radioactively labeled ocular-dominance regions, which are now seen from above instead of edge on. The actual width of the ocular-dominance regions is typically about .4 millimeter.

ble block. Whether the set of orientation slabs begins with a slab representing a vertical orientation, an oblique one or a horizontal one is completely arbitrary; so too is whether an ocular-dominance sequence begins with a left-plus-right pair of dominance slabs or a right-plus-left pair. The same thing is true for a unit crystal of sodium chloride or for any complex repetitive pattern such as is found in wallpaper.

What, then, does the visual scene really look like as it is projected onto the visual cortex? Suppose an animal fixes its gaze on some point and the only object in the visual field is a straight line above and a bit to the left of the point where the gaze is riveted. If each active cell were to light up, and if one could stand above the cortex and look down at it, what would the pattern be? To make the problem more interesting, suppose the pattern is seen by one eye only. In view of the architecture just described the pattern turns out to be not a line but merely a set of regularly spaced patches (see Figure 1.18). The reasoning can be checked directly by exposing a monkey with one eye closed to a set of vertical stripes and making a deoxyglucose autoradiograph. The resulting pattern should not be a great surprise: it is a set of regularly spaced patches, which simply represents the intersection of the two sets of column systems. Imagine the surprise and bewilderment of a little green man looking at such a version of the outside world! (See Figure 1.19.)

Why evolution has gone to the trouble of designing such an elaborate architecture is a question that

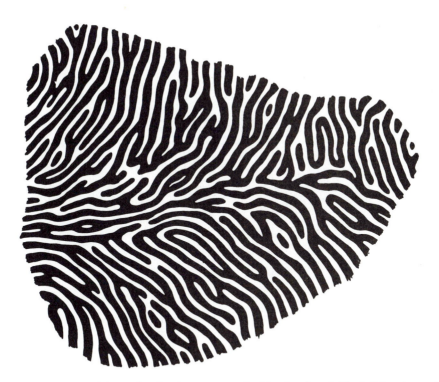

Figure 1.16 RECONSTRUCTION of the ocular-dominance pattern over the entire exposed part of the right primary visual cortex was made by the authors and Simon LeVay from a series of sections stained by a reduced-silver method he developed. The left-hand margin is at the medial edge of occipital lobe, where cortex folds downward; pattern is enlarged about six diameters.

continues to fascinate us. Perhaps the most plausible notion is that the column systems are a solution to the problem of portraying more than two dimensions on a two-dimensional surface. The cortex is dealing with at least four sets of values: two for the x and y position variables in the visual field, one for orientation and one for the different degrees of eye preference. The two surface coordinates are used up in designating field position; the other two variables are accommodated by dicing up the cortex with subdivisions so fine that one can run through a complete set of orientations or eye preferences and meanwhile have a shift in visual-field position that is small with respect to the resolution in that part of the visual world.

The strategy of subdividing the cortex with small vertical partitions is certainly not limited to the primary visual area. Such subdivisions were first seen in the somatic sensory area by Vernon B. Mountcastle of the Johns Hopkins University School of Medi-

cine about 10 years before our work in the visual area. In the somatic sensory area, as we pointed out above, the basic topography is a map of the opposite half of the body, but superimposed on that there is a two-fold system of subdivisions, with some areas where neurons respond to the movement of the joints or pressure on the skin and other areas where they respond to touch or the bending of hairs. As in the case of the visual columns, a complete set here (one area for each kind of neuron) occupies a distance of about a millimeter. These subdivisions are analogous to ocular-dominance columns in that they are determined in the first instance by inputs to the cortex (from either the left or the right eye and from either deep receptors or receptors in the upper skin layers) rather than by connections within the cortex, such as those that determine orientation selectivity and the associated system of orientation regions.

The columnar subdivisions associated with the

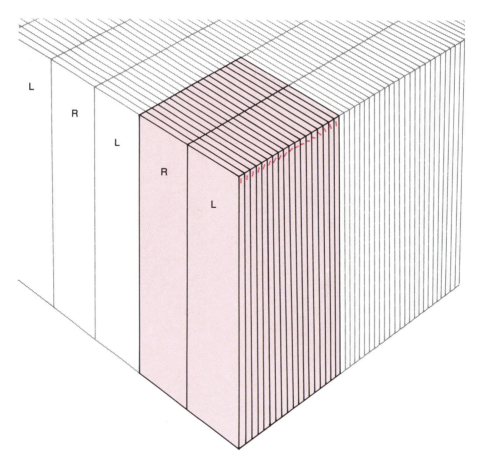

Figure 1.17 BLOCK OF CORTEX about a millimeter square and two millimeters deep (*light color*) can be considered an elementary unit of the primary visual cortex. It contains one set of orientation slabs subserving all orientations and one set of ocular-dominance slabs subserving both eyes. The pattern is reiterated throughout the primary visual area. The placing of the boundaries (at the right or the left eye, at a vertical, horizontal or oblique orientation) is arbitrary; representation of the slabs as flat planes intersecting at right angles is an oversimplification.

visual and somatic sensory systems are the best-understood ones, but there are indications of similar vertical subdivisions in some other areas: several higher visual areas, sensory parietal regions recently studied by Mountcastle and the auditory region, where Thomas J. Imig, H. O. Adrián and John F. Brugge of the University of Wisconsin Medical School and their colleagues have found subdivisions in which the two ears seem alternately to add their information or to compete.

For most of these physiologically defined systems (except the visual ones) there are so far no anatomical correlates. On the other hand, in the past few years several anatomists, notably Edward G. Jones of the Washington University School of Medicine and Nauta and Patricia Goldman at MIT, have shown that connections from one region of the cortex to another (for example from the somatic sensory area on one side to the corresponding area on the other side) terminate in patches that have a regular periodicity of about a millimeter. Here the columns are evident morphologically, but one has

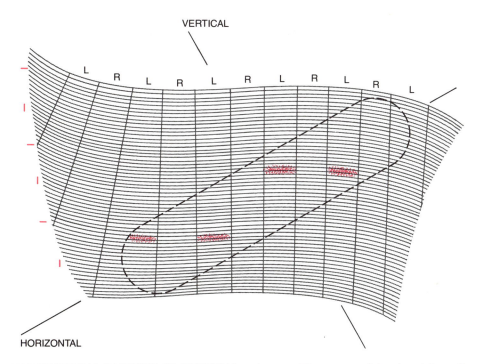

Figure 1.18 HYPOTHETICAL PATTERN OF CORTICAL ACTIVITY that might result from stimulation of the left eye with a single short horizontal line, placed in the upper left quadrant of the visual field, is shown by the colored patches on a diagram of an area of the right cortex, seen face on. The area receiving input from the object in the visual field is indicated by the broken black line. If ocular-dominance and orientation columns are arrayed as shown, activated cells will be those that respond optimally to approximately horizontal stimuli from the left eye.

no idea of the physiological interpretation. It is clear, however, that fine periodic subdivisions are a very general feature of the cerebral cortex. Indeed, Mountcastle's original observation of that feature may be said to supply a fourth profound insight into cortical organization.

It would surely be wrong to assume that this account of the visual cortex in any way exhausts the subject. Color, movement and stereoscopic depth are probably all dealt with in the cortex, but to what extent or how is still not clear. There are indications from work we and others have done on depth and from work on color by Semir Zeki of University College London that higher cortical visual areas to which the primary area projects directly or indi-

rectly may be specialized to handle these variables, but we are a long way from knowing what the handling involves.

What happens beyond the primary visual area, and how is the information on orientation exploited at later stages? Is one to imagine ultimately finding a cell that responds specifically to some very particular item? (Usually one's grandmother is selected as the particular item, for reasons that escape us.) Our answer is that we doubt there is such a cell, but we have no good alternative to offer. To speculate broadly on how the brain may work is fortunately not the only course open to investigators. To explore the brain is more fun and seems to be more profitable.

There was a time, not so long ago, when one looked at the millions of neurons in the various

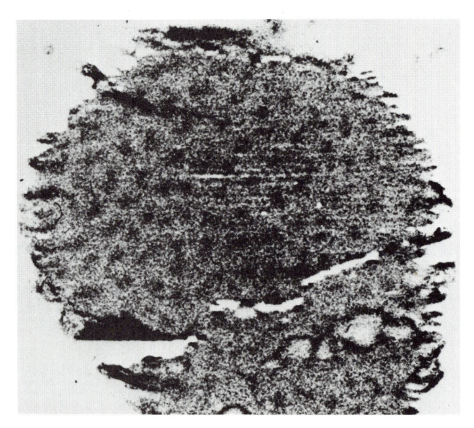

Figure 1.19 ACTUAL PATTERN of cortical activity was elicited by exposing only the left eye to a set of vertical stripes. The deoxyglucose autoradiograph is of a tangential section in the outer layers of the cortex. The pattern of regularly spaced dark patches of radioactivity represents intersection of ocular-dominance and orientation systems. Magnification is about eight diameters.

layers of the cortex and wondered if anyone would ever have any idea of their function. Did they all work in parallel, like the cells of the liver or the kidney, achieving their objectives by pure bulk, or were they each doing something special? For the visual cortex the answer seems now to be known in broad outline: Particular stimuli turn neurons on or off; groups of neurons do indeed perform particular transformations. It seems reasonable to think that if the secrets of a few regions such as this one can be unlocked, other regions will also in time give up their secrets.

Negative Aftereffects in Visual Perception

You will see one if you stare at a waterfall for a short time and then look away; the surrounding scene will seem to move slowly upward. The study of such illusions yields information on perceptual systems.

• • •

Olga Eizner Favreau and Michael C. Corballis
December, 1976

It is a common experience to look at a bright light and to find that a dark image of the object remains in the visual field for some time afterward. The phenomenon is called a negative afterimage (negative because the object was bright and the image is dark). A similar phenomenon can be experienced by staring for several minutes at something that is moving in a uniform direction, as a waterfall does, and then turning the gaze away; the surrounding scene will appear to drift slowly in the opposite direction. This is a negative aftereffect. Afterimages and aftereffects are illusions, reminding one that the senses are sometimes imperfect mediators between the external world and one's perception of it. The study of such illusions is valuable in psychology for the clues they provide to how the sense organs and the nervous system function in processing information.

Afterimages and aftereffects are encountered in a variety of forms. For example, afterimages of colored objects appear in colors that are complementary to the colors of the objects. If you stare at a patch of green for a minute or so and then look at a blank field, you can expect to see a reddish patch of the same shape (see Figure 2.1).

In addition to motion aftereffects of the kind evoked by watching a waterfall one can experience figural aftereffects. For example, if you look at a line that is tilted about 15 degrees from the vertical, a line that is actually vertical may appear to be tilted in the opposite direction (see Figure 2.2). A related aftereffect can be observed if you look at a curved line for a time; a straight line then seems to curve the other way (see Figure 2.3).

Aftereffects are by no means limited to vision. If someone is blindfolded and then runs a finger back and forth along a curved rod, a straight rod will seem to be curved the other way. Similarly, as has been demonstrated by Stuart M. Anstis of York University, if one listens repeatedly to a tone that increases in intensity, a tone of constant intensity is likely to sound as though it is decreasing in intensity. Here we shall focus on visual aftereffects, since they have been the most intensively examined.

A number of investigators in the 19th century thought motion aftereffects might be related to movements of the eyes. Exposure to a moving pattern induces the eyes to follow the motion of the pattern. If the eyes tend to persist in the same pat-

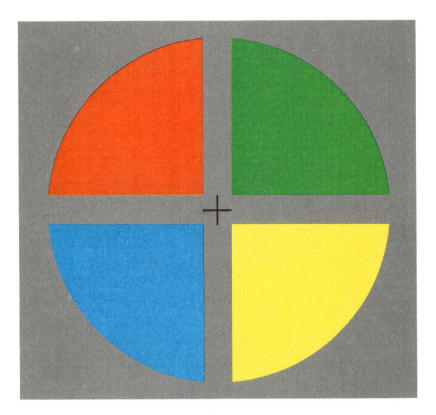

Figure 2.1 NEGATIVE AFTER-IMAGE is the simplest kind of negative aftereffect. Here the afterimage will appear in the color that is complementary to the color you look at. If you fix your gaze on the cross at the center of the colors for about a minute and then look at the gray field at the bottom of the page, you should see patches that are in the complementary colors of the original: the green, yellow, blue and red will be replaced respectively by red, blue, yellow and green.

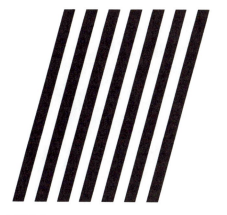 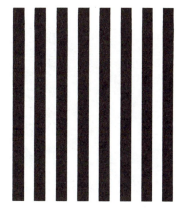

Figure 2.2 TILT AFTEREFFECT appears when one has looked steadily for a minute or more at the tilted lines.

Thereafter lines that are actually vertical will seem to tilt in the opposite direction.

tern of scanning when the movement is no longer there, a stationary pattern might then seem to move in the opposite direction.

In 1850, however, this hypothesis was discredited by the Belgian physicist Joseph Plateau on the basis of work with rotating spirals. Such a spiral appears either to expand or to contract, depending on the direction of rotation. Plateau found that if one watches an expanding spiral for a few minutes, a stationary spiral then seems to contract; conversely, a contracting spiral induces an aftereffect of expansion. The spiral aftereffect cannot be explained simply in terms of eye movements, because both ex-

pansion and contraction consist of movement in all directions at once (see Figure 2.4).

Another explanation for aftereffects is the concept of normalization proposed by J. J. Gibson of Cornell University. He argued that a prolonged exposure to a stimulus that deviates in some way from an established norm might serve to redefine the norm. For example, an exposure to a line that is tilted slightly from the vertical might induce the observer to recalibrate his conception of the vertical toward the line. A truly vertical line would then be seen as being tilted in the other direction. This hypothesis may be partly correct, but it cannot easily

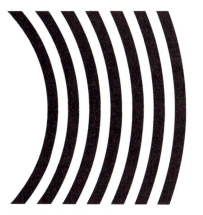 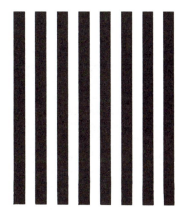

Figure 2.3 CURVE AFTEREFFECT results from looking at curved lines for several minutes, moving the eyes only

along the central portion. The straight lines will then appear to curve the opposite way.

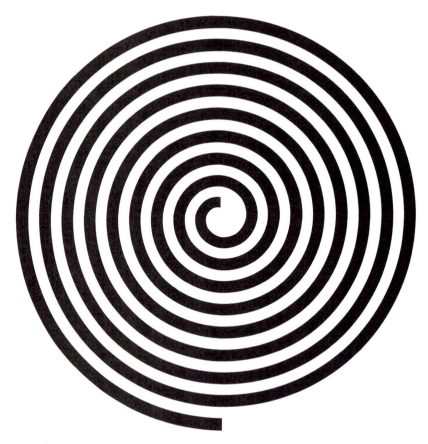

Figure 2.4 SPIRAL AFTEREFFECT is caused by putting a spiral on a turntable and rotating it at 33 1/3 revolutions per minute. When the spiral is stopped, it seems to move in the other direction.

account for aftereffects that arise when no obvious norm is involved. As Donald E. Mitchell and Darwin W. Muir of Dalhousie University have shown, the tilt aftereffect induced with a stimulus of oblique lines is similar in both magnitude and direction to the aftereffects induced with vertical and horizontal lines.

In recent years attempts to understand visual aftereffects have drawn increasingly on concepts derived from the growing body of knowledge of the neurophysiology of the visual system. Although most of this work is based on recordings made with microelectrodes from individual neurons, or nerve cells, in the visual system of such animals as cats and monkeys, a number of psychologists have been quick to extrapolate the findings to human vision. The exchange has also gone the other way: concepts derived from work on aftereffects in human beings preceded fundamental discoveries in the neurophysiology of vision in other primates. We hope to convey something of the flavor of this exchange between disciplines.

Light reaching the eye is focused by the lens to form a two-dimensional image on the retina. Light-sensitive receptors there convert the image into a spatial pattern of neural impulses. The impulses are transmitted from the receptors to a layer of neurons called bipolar cells and then to another layer called retinal ganglion cells. Fibers from the retinal ganglion cells make up the optic nerve, which carries the neural information from the retina to the brain.

Negative and complementary afterimages probably depend largely on the properties of cells in the retina. It is easy to demonstrate that an afterimage moves about as one moves one's eyes and that its location is perfectly correlated with the position of the eyes; it is as though the afterimage were painted on the retina. In contrast, objects actually present in the visual field appear to remain fixed if one moves one's eyes. These observations hold only for normal, voluntary eye movements. The situation is reversed if one moves an eye passively, as by pressing at the corner of the eye with a finger; then objects in the real world appear to move but an afterimage remains motionless. Both kinds of observation show that afterimages are formed at a level of processing preceding the one where the perceived location of objects in space is "corrected" for voluntary eye movements.

It is also easy to show that afterimages do not transfer from one eye to the other. The reader can verify this finding by looking at the top half of Figure 2.1 for about 40 seconds with a hand over one eye. The afterimage will then be visible against a plain surface, such as at the bottom half of Figure 2.1, only to the exposed eye.

One can explain these phenomena by supposing cells in the retina, including the receptors, become temporarily fatigued or adapted after a long stimulation. According to this reasoning, if one looks at, say, a white patch, cells responsive to white light become less responsive, leaving an impression of a dark patch if the gaze is shifted to a uniform field. Complementary afterimages (red following green, for example) can be explained in a similar way.

Neurons beyond the receptors may also contribute to afterimages. They include the bipolar and ganglion cells in the retina and possibly cells in the lateral geniculate nucleus, a relay station in the brain that receives its input directly from the retinal ganglion cells. Among the retinal ganglion cells and the lateral geniculate cells are cells that typically exhibit what is termed "opponent process" organization, meaning that a cell increases its normal rate of firing in response to one color but decreases it in response to the complementary color. Opponent-process cells might contribute to afterimages in two ways. Suppose one views a uniform green field for a period of time. The cells that fire at an increased rate for green (they are called green-on, red-off cells) may become fatigued, so that if one subsequently views a uniform white field, the reduced firing of these cells is interpreted as redness. Conversely,

red-on, green-off cells would be depressed while one was looking at a green field and might subsequently "rebound" to enhance the impression of redness.

Whereas afterimages depend on the fatigue of cells in the early stages of visual processing, figural and motion aftereffects appear to depend on properties of neurons at a higher level, perhaps in the visual cortex. The study of such aftereffects was greatly stimulated by the pioneering discoveries of David H. Hubel and Tosten N. Wiesel of the Harvard Medical School on the properties of neurons in the visual cortex of the cat brain [see Chapter 1, "Brain Mechanisms of Vision," by David H. Hubel and Torsten N. Wiesel; see also "The Visual Cortex of the Brain," by David H. Hubel; SCIENTIFIC AMERICAN, November, 1963; Offprint 168]. Hubel and Wiesel found cells that they classified hierarchically as simple, complex and hypercomplex. Simple cells respond to edges, slits or lines. The edge, slit or line must be precisely located and oriented in the visual field to cause a given cell to fire at the maximum rate. Although location is not so critical for complex and hypercomplex cells, they have the added characteristic of responding maximally when the preferred stimulus is in motion in a direction perpendicular to its orientation. Many of these cells are also directionally selective in that they respond to motion in one direction but not to motion in the opposite direction.

In 1961, two years after the first report by Hubel and Wiesel, N. Stuart Sutherland, who is now at the University of Sussex, suggested that cortical cells of the kind described by the Harvard workers might underlie aftereffects of motion and orientation. His explanation, like the one we have described for afterimages, invoked the concept of neural fatigue. According to Sutherland, the perception of the orientation of a line would involve a kind of averaging of the activity of all the line detectors that respond to the line. If one looks at, say, a vertical line, the neurons most sensitive to verticalness are the most active and there is no overall bias due to the activity of cells sensitive to other orientations. The decision about the orientation of the line therefore corresponds to reality.

Now suppose the observer looks for some time at a line that is tilted 15 degrees clockwise (see Figure 2.2). Line detectors maximally sensitive to the 15-degree line become fatigued, so that when the observer looks at the vertical line, the balance of activity is shifted counterclockwise away from the vertical. A similar process could underlie motion aftereffects.

The recognition that single cells in the cat's brain are simultaneously sensitive to more than one specific feature of environmental stimuli, such as orientation and brightness, introduced the possibility of discovering aftereffects with multiple components. The possibility was first realized by Celeste McCollough, then at Oberlin College. She reasoned that human beings probably have line detectors similar to the ones found in cats and that since people, unlike cats, also have color vision it might not be unreasonable to suppose that human line detectors are specialized for color as well as for orientation. If they are, one might be able to demonstrate aftereffects that depend on both the orientation and the color of lines.

McCollough accomplished the demonstration in the following way. Subjects looked at grids of horizontal green and black lines alternating every few seconds with grids of vertical orange and black lines (see Figure 2.5). After about 10 minutes they were shown grids of horizontal and of vertical white and black lines. The horizontal grids appeared to have a faint orange color and the vertical grids were tinged with green (see Figure 2.6). This result can be described as an orientation-contingent color aftereffect; it is generally known as the McCollough effect.

It is unlikely that the McCollough effect is retinal in origin. For one thing it is clear that the perceived colors are not simply complementary afterimages, since either color can be seen in the same retinal location, depending only on the orientation of the lines in the grid. Moreover, it is not necessary to gaze fixedly at the figures in order to get the McCollough effect.

Another aspect of the McCollough effect that differentiates it from simple afterimages is its extreme persistence. With an adaptation period of 10 or 15 minutes the effect may still be visible days or even weeks later. Because of these properties it is generally believed that the mechanisms responsible for the McCollough effect are localized in the visual cortex of the cerebrum. Three years after McCollough's discovery Hubel and Wiesel reported that the visual cortex of the monkey does in fact contain neurons sensitive to both the orientation and the color of a stimulus.

Other reports of contingent aftereffects have followed McCollough's work. Norva Hepler of McGill University and Charles F. Stromeyer and R. J. W. Mansfield of Harvard University independently discovered that color aftereffects can be made contingent on the direction of motion of a pattern. For example, if an observer alternately watches a spiral rotating clockwise in green light and counterclockwise in red light, a black-and-white spiral may subsequently appear pinkish if it is rotated clockwise and greenish if it is rotated counterclockwise.

We and Victor F. Emerson, working at McGill, discovered that it is possible to induce the converse of this contingency. (The finding was also reported by Anstis and John E. W. Mayhew.) After watching a green clockwise spiral alternating with a red counterclockwise spiral observers report that a stationary spiral appears to move briefly counterclockwise when it is green and clockwise when it is red. This is a color-contingent motion aftereffect. Like the motion-contingent color aftereffect, it is long-lasting, that is, although it is brief for any one exposure to a colored spiral, it can reappear when the spiral is looked at again. Both the color-contingent motion aftereffect and the motion-contingent color aftereffect can reappear if an observer is shown the test patterns 24 hours after adaptation.

The evidence we have reviewed so far seems to support the view that aftereffects depend on the properties of feature detectors that bear a close functional resemblance to the neurons described by Hubel and Wiesel. Nevertheless, investigators in both neurophysiology and human perception have recently sought to prove the existence of detectors that respond to more integrated properties of the visual display. Indeed, some workers now believe the neurons studied by Hubel and Wiesel do not function simply as edge, slit or line detectors but also contribute to an analysis of the spatial frequencies (the spacing of more or less regularly repeating elements) in the total display. It has been found that individual neurons in the visual cortex of the cat respond selectively to sinusoidal gratings (parallel bars having a brightness that varies in a sinusoidal manner across the grating) only within a narrow range of spatial frequencies [see "Contrast and Spatial Frequency," by Fergus W. Campbell and Lamberto Maffei; SCIENTIFIC AMERICAN, November, 1974].

A number of aftereffects can be attributed to detectors of spatial frequency. For example, Colin

Blakemore and Peter Sutton of the University of Cambridge discovered that if one looks at a striped pattern for some minutes and then views a grating with the same orientation but slightly narrower bars, the bars seem even narrower and more closely spaced than they really are. Conversely, broader bars seem broader (see Figure 2.7).

The explanation proposed by Blakemore and Sutton was similar to the one advanced by Sutherland to explain tilt and motion aftereffects. They suggested that a grating of a particular frequency arouses activity in a subpopulation of frequency-detecting neurons. The distribution of activity is averaged to provide a perceptual impression of what the displayed frequency is. Preadaptation to some other spatial frequency would have depressed the activity of neurons sensitive to that frequency and so would skew the distribution away from the distribution normally evoked by the displayed pattern.

Color aftereffects can also be made contingent on spatial frequency. W. J. Lovegrove and Ray F. Over of the University of Queensland had subjects watch a vertical grating of one spatial frequency in red light alternating with a vertical grating of a different spatial frequency in green light. Afterward a black-and-white test grating of the first frequency appeared greenish and a grating of the second frequency appeared pinkish. Color aftereffects occurred, however, only if the frequency of one grating was at least twice that of the other and if the frequency of at least one grating was higher than three cycles per degree of visual angle. Lovegrove and Over suggested that their results could be explained in terms of the adaptation of neural units tuned for both color and spatial frequency.

A useful way to check on the location in the visual system of the neurons responsible for aftereffects is to test for interactions of the eyes. For example, one can induce an aftereffect in one eye and then ask whether the observer sees it when he looks with the other eye. Neurons in the visual pathway from the retina to the visual cortex are driven by one eye up to and including the lateral geniculate nucleus. In the visual cortex some neurons are driven monocularly (by an input to one eye only) and others are driven binocularly (by an input to either eye). Most of the cells in the superior colliculus (another part of the visual-processing sys-

tem) are driven binocularly (see Figure 2.8). Hence if an aftereffect is observed to transfer from one eye to the other, one can infer that it is mediated by cells in either the visual cortex or the superior colliculus. Since neurons in the superior colliculus appear to be sensitive mainly to motion, however, their role (if they have one) would be confined to motion aftereffects.

It has generally been found that figural and motion aftereffects, unlike afterimages, do transfer from one eye to the other, although their strength is reduced in the process. These aftereffects are therefore probably mediated by both monocularly and binocularly driven neurons. In the eye that was exposed to the adapting pattern both kinds of neurons would mediate the effect. In the other eye, however, only the neurons driven binocularly would be involved, which accounts for the reduction in strength.

Contingent aftereffects where one of the components is color apparently do not transfer from one eye to the other. This finding suggested that they may be mediated by monocularly driven neurons. Some evidence indicates, however, that this hypothesis may not be altogether correct. Experiments conducted by T. R. Vidyasagar of the University of Manchester have indicated that orientation-contingent color aftereffects can involve neurons that require an input to both eyes. Such neurons are binocular, but they could not mediate an interocular transfer. It seems possible that other contingent aftereffects may also involve binocular neurons of this type.

Gerald M. Murch of Portland State University has demonstrated that the color and motion components of an aftereffect can be dissociated. He has also shown that the motion component transfers from one eye to the other and the color component does not. Murch's procedure involved an adaptation phase and a test phase. In the adaptation phase he presented to the right eye a spiral whose motion was alternated between clockwise and counterclockwise, and at the same time he presented to the left eye the contingent color, alternately red and green. In the test phase the observer looked at stationary red or green spirals with first one eye and then the other. The contingent aftereffect (clockwise movement of the green spiral and counterclockwise movement of the red one) was reported only when the observer used his left eye. The adaptation to motion thus transferred from one eye to the other

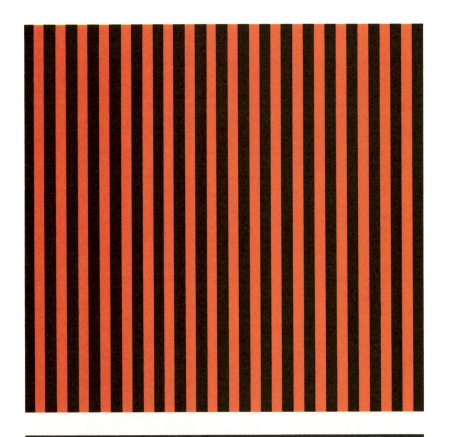

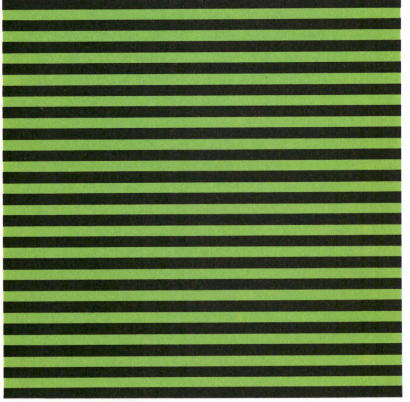

Figure 2.5 CONTINGENT AF-TEREFFECT is demonstrated by these two grids and the pattern in Figure 2.6. Look alternately at one grid and then the other for about 10 seconds each for 10 minutes. Then look at the pattern in Figure 2.6. Its horizontal lines should appear reddish and its vertical lines greenish. If the page is turned 90 degrees, the color relations reverse. The phenomenon is termed an orientation-contingent color aftereffect.

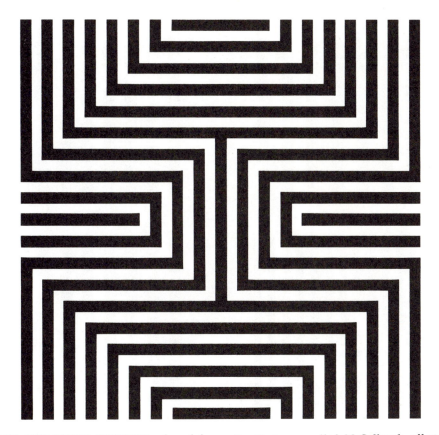

Figure 2.6 BLACK-AND-WHITE PATTERN, viewed in conjunction with grids in Figure 2.5, produces the orientation-contingent color aftereffect. Such multiple-component aftereffects are called McCollough effects after Celeste McCollough, who discovered them.

but the information about the contingent colors did not.

Murch's elegant experiment raises a general question about the nature of contingent aftereffects. Until recently it had been widely assumed that they are due solely to the adaptation of "multiple duty" neurons tuned to the different components, such as color and orientation, that underlie the aftereffects. Murch and other workers have questioned this assumption, suggesting instead that the contingency may depend on associative connections between different classes of neurons, each type tuned to a single component of the visual experience. Although Murch's experiment does not rule out the participation of multiple-duty neurons in the mediation of contingent aftereffects, it does introduce the possibility that such aftereffects can also be me-

diated by associations among previously independent neurons.

The possibility that contingent aftereffects may depend on the formation of associative connections rather than (or perhaps in addition to) fatigue has been suggested for another reason, namely the persistence of many contingent aftereffects. As we have mentioned, they can be detected days or even weeks after the adaptation period. We know of no neurophysiological evidence that fatigue or the adaptation of single neurons ever persists for such a long time.

Indeed, the persistence may not be confined to contingent aftereffects, although the question of whether or not an aftereffect is contingent is sometimes a fine point. Richard F. Masland of McGill showed that features of the spiral aftereffect can

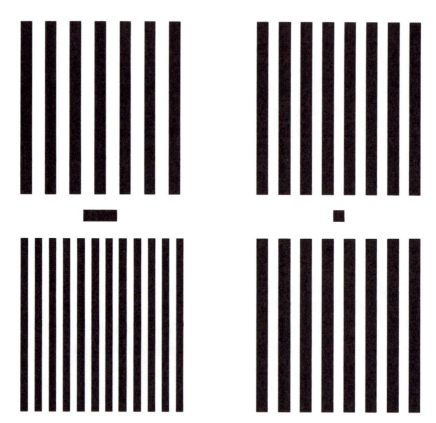

Figure 2.7 SPATIAL VARIATIONS can cause aftereffects, apparently because neurons are sensitive to spatial frequencies, the spacing of regular features of what you are looking at. First, look at the two sets of vertical bars at the right to establish that they are the same. Then move your eyes back and forth along the horizontal bar between the two sets of vertical bars on the left for several minutes. When you shift your gaze to the horizontal bar between the vertical grids at the right, the spatial frequency of the grid at the top will appear to be higher than that of the grid at the bottom. If the figure is turned upside down, the spatial relations will then reverse.

persist for as long as 24 hours. One of us (Favreau) has found that it may still be present a week later. The decrease in magnitude of the spiral aftereffect is rapid during the first few minutes, but thereafter the rate of decease is markedly slower. For this reason Masland suggested that the aftereffect has two components: a rapidly decaying component directly due to the adaptation of motion detectors and a more slowly decaying, more persistent component caused by the conditioned adaptation of the detectors. In conditioned adaptation, although the motion detectors would not remain fatigued for the entire period during which the aftereffect persists, the spiral configuration, having become associated with fatigue, could cause the detectors to return to a state resembling fatigue.

Although the concept of conditioned adaptation or fatigue could be useful in explaining the long-term persistence of negative aftereffects, it presents a stumbling block. If the various attributes of the inducing stimulus, such as spiral configuration and clockwise motion, become associated with one another, one would expect to obtain positive aftereffects rather than negative ones. Thus, for example, a stationary spiral would appear to rotate in the direction in which the spiral was previously seen rotating and a colorless vertical grating employed to test for the McCollough effect would appear green if the vertical orientation had been paired with green. The striking feature of negative aftereffects, however, is that when two attributes are combined in a stimulus, one of them subsequently becomes associated

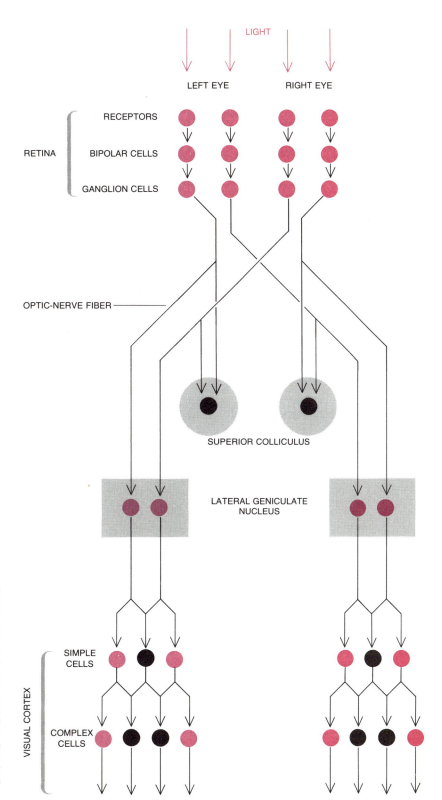

Figure 2.8 VISUAL SYSTEM is depicted schematically to show the flow of information. The neurons, or nerve cells, represented in color are driven by only one eye, whereas the ones shown in black are driven by both eyes. Hence if an aftereffect that has been induced in one eye is observed to transfer to the other eye, one can infer that it is mediated by cells either in the visual cortex of the brain or in the superior colliculus. Afterimages, in contrast to aftereffects, do not transfer from one eye to the other, so that they evidently originate in early stages of visual processing.

LIGHT

LEFT EYE   RIGHT EYE

RECEPTORS

RETINA   BIPOLAR CELLS

GANGLION CELLS

OPTIC-NERVE FIBER

SUPERIOR COLLICULUS

LATERAL GENICULATE NUCLEUS

VISUAL CORTEX

SIMPLE CELLS

COMPLEX CELLS

with an opposite quality of the other (movement in the other direction, the complementary color and so on).

It is plausible that fatigue could become associated with aspects of the adapting stimulus, since it is known that the processes of fatigue start operating as soon as one looks at a stimulus. When one views something that is constantly moving, the perceived velocity decreases. When one looks at a colored surface, the color appears to become desaturated. (The reader can verify this relation by looking at one of the colored patches in Figure 2.1. If half of the patch is obscured by a piece of gray paper that is removed after about 30 seconds, the part of the patch that was covered appears to be brighter than the part that was exposed.)

We have now examined two possible explanations of negative aftereffects: fatigue and conditioned fatigue. Possibly they both play a role. Masland's work on the spiral aftereffect showed that it has two components. One of us (Favreau) has conducted experiments that suggest a further dissociation of the short- and long-term components of this aftereffect. The simple aftereffect is observable immediately after one looks at a spiral, and it also decreases steadily in strength. The color-contingent spiral aftereffect is not seen immediately and does not reach full strength for several minutes. The finding suggests that during an exposure to spirals of alternating motion and colors, visual units sensitive to both directions of motion may become fatigued and hence prevent the rapid appearance of a motion aftereffect. As the fatigue wears off, the effects of mechanisms underlying the color contingency may be revealed.

If contingent aftereffects do depend on the formation of associative connections between visual units, the question arises of how such connections are established. One possibility is that information from different sets of feature-extracting neurons converges in a mutually interactive way at a higher level of visual processing. The interaction (between, say, color and motion) would be recorded by a relative adaptation across a bank of neurons at the higher level. Thereafter the activation of this system by either of the original sets of neurons could recreate the impression of adaptation in the other set, thereby yielding the appropriate negative aftereffect.

This account still relies on the notion of adaptation, or habituation, of neurons. These hypothetical neurons, however, are at least removed from the feature-analyzing neurons that have been studied intensively and have not been observed to exhibit long-term adaptation effects. Neurons of this kind, which store patterns of interaction by means of long-term habituation, may play a rather general role in learning and memory

COLOR AND LIGHTNESS

. . .

The Retinex Theory of Color Vision

A retina-and-cortex system (retinex) may treat a color as a code for a three-part report from the retina, independent of the flux of radiant energy but correlated with the reflectance of objects.

. . .

Edwin H. Land
December, 1977

The scientific tradition of simplifying the conditions of an experiment has left us until recently without a satisfactory explanation of how the eye sees color in everyday life. Paradoxically the modern technology of color photography has reinforced the belief that the colors discerned by Newton in the spectrum are, with minor qualifications, the colors of the world around us. We know, for example, that if we use daylight color film when we take a picture in the light shed by an ordinary tungsten-filament lamp, the picture will turn out to have a strong reddish cast. That, we say, is because the rays from the tungsten filament are too "red," never asking how we ourselves can move constantly in and out of tungsten-lit worlds without experiencing any change in the color of familiar objects: apples, lemons, strawberries, bread, human faces (the tones of which are so hard to get right on a television screen).

How, then, does the eye deal with the excess of "red" in a tungsten-lit room? As I hope to demonstrate in this chapter, the eye, in determining color, never perceives the extra red because it does not depend on the flux of radiant energy reaching it. The eye has evolved to see the world in unchanging colors, regardless of always unpredictable, shifting and uneven illumination. How the eye achieves this remarkable feat has fascinated me for many years.

In 1959 I described in an article for SCIENTIFIC AMERICAN, a series of experiments in which a scene created by the superposition of two black-and-white transparencies, one projected through a red filter and the other projected without a filter (that is, in white light), conveys to the eye nearly the gamut of colors present in the original scene [see "Experiments in Color Vision," by Edwin H. Land; SCIENTIFIC AMERICAN, May 1959]. To produce such "red-and-white" images the picture projected through the red filter is taken through a red filter and the picture projected in white light is taken through a green filter. It would be expected that the superposed image on the projection screen could generate only red, white and various shades of pink. Actually one sees a picture remarkably similar to the full-color photograph reproduced in Figure 3.1. (Black and white images of the same still life taken with four different film-filter combinations are shown in Figure 3.2.) In the red-and-white photographic projection peppers are green, radishes and strawberries are red, the orange is orange, the lemon and ba-

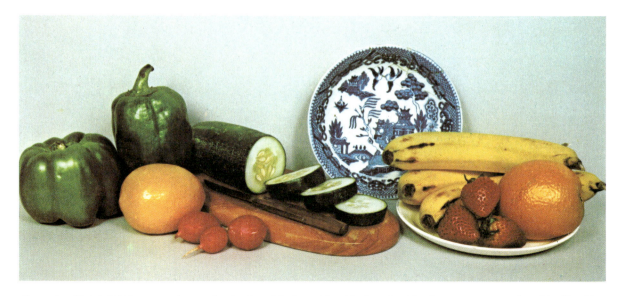

Figure 3.1 STILL LIFE was used to make the four black-and-white images presented in Figure 3.2. The reproduction of the still life was made by conventional processes of color photography and photoengraving to show the reader what the colors of the original objects in the scene were. The black-and-white images were made with film-filter combinations that closely duplicate the separate wavelength sensitivities of the four systems of photoreceptors in the retina of the eye: the three systems of cone cells and the hypersensitive system of rod cells.

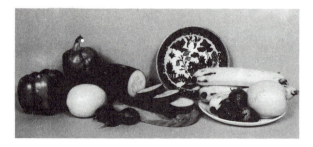

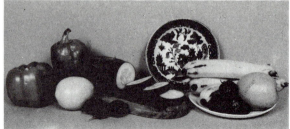

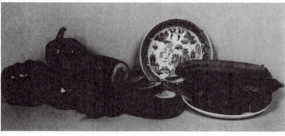

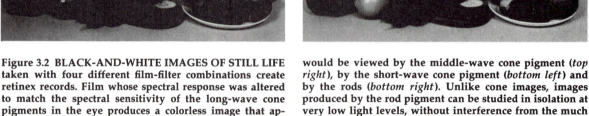

Figure 3.2 BLACK-AND-WHITE IMAGES OF STILL LIFE taken with four different film-filter combinations create retinex records. Film whose spectral response was altered to match the spectral sensitivity of the long-wave cone pigments in the eye produces a colorless image that approximates the image produced by the long-wave cones by themselves (*top left*). The same scene is produced as it would be viewed by the middle-wave cone pigment (*top right*), by the short-wave cone pigment (*bottom left*) and by the rods (*bottom right*). Unlike cone images, images produced by the rod pigment can be studied in isolation at very low light levels, without interference from the much less sensitive cone systems.

nanas are pale yellow, the wood cutting board and knife handle are brown and the design on the plate is blue.

The challenge presented by our early red-and-white experiments led us step by step over a 20-year period to an explanation of how the visual system is able to extract reliable color information from the world around us, a world in which virtually every scene is lighted unevenly, in which the spectral composition of the radiation falling on a scene can vary enormously and in which illumination as brief as a lightning flash suffices for the accurate identification of color. If the nature of the responses of the photoreceptors in the retina of the eye even approximated what most of us were taught in school, functioning primarily as intensity-level meters with peaks in three different parts of the spectrum, we would be continually confusing one color with another. An object that looked yellow in one part of our field of view might look green or gray or even red when moved to a different part of the field. The fact remains that objects retain their color identity under a great variety of lighting conditions. This constancy is not a minor second-order effect but is so fundamental as to call for a new description of how we see color.

The visual pigments are photosensitive molecules that respond to a wide band of light frequencies. The three pigments in the cone cells of the retina cover the visible spectrum in three broad, overlapping curves. The pigment with a peak sensitivity at a wavelength of 440 nanometers responds in some degree to the entire lower-frequency half of the visible spectrum. Each of the other two pigments responds to almost two-thirds of the visible spectrum, the two being offset at their peaks by barely 30 nanometers, with their peak sensitivities located at 535 and 565 nanometers (see Figure 3.3).

In this discussion the names of colors—"red," "green," "blue" and so on—will be reserved for the color sensation we have when we look at the world around us. In short, only our eyes can categorize the color of objects: spectrophotometers cannot. This point is not a trivial one because many people viewing some of our experiments for the first time will identify something as being red or green but will then ask, as if their eyes were being fooled, "What color is it really?" The answer is that the eye is not being fooled. It is functioning exactly as it must with involuntary reliability to see constant colors in a world illuminated by shifting and unpredictable fluxes of radiant energy.

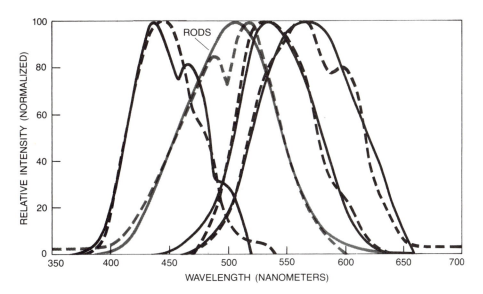

Figure 3.3 NORMALIZED SPECTRAL SENSITIVITIES OF FOUR VISUAL PIGMENTS (solid lines) span the visual spectrum in overlapping curves. Curve that peaks at about 500 nanometers corresponds to sensitivity of rod pigment. Other three curves represent cone pigments. Broken lines show sensitivities of the film-filter combinations that were selected to match the sensitivities of the four retinal pigments and used to make the black-and-white retinex records in Figure 3.2. Cone curves are adapted from work of Paul Brown and George Wald of Harvard University. The rod curve is standard scotopic luminosity curve.

Since I believe the study of color in fully colored images is best begun by examining images that are completely devoid of and completely uncomplicated by the experience of color, let me describe that experience in some detail. The hypersensitive system based on the rod cells in the retina functions at light levels as much as 1,000 times weaker than the systems based on the cone cells do, so that it is possible to answer the interesting question: What colors will one see if only the rod system is activated? One procedure is to put on a pair of tightly fitting goggles equipped with neutral-density filters that reduce the incident light by a factor of 30,000. After one has worn the goggles for about half an hour objects in a room illuminated to the typical level of 20 foot-candles will become visible. The effective illumination in the room will thus be 1/1,500 foot-candle. As one looks around the room the familiar colored objects will be seen devoid of color, exhibiting instead a range of lightnesses from white to black, much as they would appear in a black-and-white photograph taken through a green color-separation filter. In other words, the reds will appear very dark, the greens lighter, the blues dark, the whites light and the blacks very dark.

In this colorless world one finds that the nature of the image is not determined by the flux of radiant energy reaching the eye. The illumination can easily be arranged so that there is more flux from a region that continues to look very dark than there is from a region that continues to look very light, whether these regions are three-dimensional objects or artifacts contrived with a montage of dark and light pieces of paper. The paradox immediately arises that each of the objects, the pieces of paper for example, whether dark or light or in between, maintains its lightness without significant change as it is moved around the room into regions of higher or lower flux. Light papers will be seen as being light and dark papers simultaneously as being dark, even with the same flux coming from each of them to the eye. Strong gradients of flux across the field will be apparent only weakly, if at all.

Furthermore, in an intricate collage of areas of various lightnesses, sizes and shapes, the lightness of a given element does not change visibly as it is relocated in any part of the collage and associated with a new arbitrary surround. When a small area is totally surrounded by a large area, the lightness of the small area will change somewhat depending on whether the large area is darker or lighter than the small one. In general, however, the impressive fact is that the lightness of a given area is not appreciably modified by the immediately surrounding areas, nor is it modified by the still larger areas surrounding them.

Although I have been describing a colorless world as it is seen by the hypersensitive receptors of rod vision, all the observations about the stability of lightness values can readily be reproduced with a montage of white, black and gray papers viewed at ordinary light levels. If, for example, a square of matte-surface black paper or, better still, black velvet is placed at one side of such a montage and a square of white paper is placed at the opposite side several feet away, with an assortment of light and dark papers scattered in between, one can place a strong light source close enough to the black square so that it sends more radiant energy to the eye than the white square, remote from the light; yet the black square will continue to look black and the white square white. In fact, with the montage still strongly illuminated from one side either the black square or the white one can be moved to any other part of the montage without a significant change in its appearance.

This remarkable ability of the eye to discover lightness values independent of flux, so convincingly demonstrated when only a single photoreceptor system is operating, is the rock on which a satisfactory description of color vision can be built. The first response of the visual system is for the receptors to absorb the light falling on the retina. Whereas the initial signal produced in the outer segment of the receptor cell is apparently proportional to the light flux absorbed by the visual pigment, the final comprehensive response of the visual system is "lightness," which shows little or no relation to the light flux absorbed by the visual pigment.

The processing of fluxes to generate lightnesses could occur in the retina, or in the cerebral cortex, or partially in both. Since we are uncertain of the location of the mechanisms that mediate these processes, I have coined the term retinex (a combination of retina and cortex) to describe the ensemble of biological mechanisms that convert flux into a pattern of lightnesses. I shall therefore use the term throughout this chapter in referring to these biological mechanisms. I shall also reserve the term lightness to mean the sensation produced by a biological system. Although the rods can be stimulated at light intensities below the cone threshold, the cones cannot be stimulated without exciting the rods. For cones we must study the lightness images produced by each individual set of receptors using retinex photography, as I shall explain below, or learn the properties of lightness images from model calculations based on spectroradiometric measurements.

Now that we know that at low light levels an isolated receptor system generates an image in terms of lightness that is completely free of color, might it be possible to bring one of the cone systems into operation along with the hypersensitive system, so that only the completely colorless system and one other were functioning? This two-receptor experiment has been carried out and provides a powerful confirmation of the ideas derived from all our binary work with red-and-white images and subsequent ternary studies with multicolored displays seen under various illuminants. The experiment, rapidly becoming a classic, was devised by my colleagues John J. McCann and Jeanne L. Benton.

McCann and Benton illuminated a color display with a narrow wave band of light at 550 nanometers. The light level was raised just above the amount needed to make the display visible to the dark-adapted eye, thus ensuring that only the hypersensitive system was operating. They then added a second narrow-band illuminant at 656 nanometers, with its level adjusted so that it was just sufficient to activate the long-wave receptor system but not the middle-wave system. Under these conditions only two receptor systems, namely the rods and the long-wave cones, were receiving enough light to function (see Figure 3.4).

The resulting image exhibited a remarkable range of color, enabling an observer to assign to each area in the display the same color name it would have if it were illuminated above the cone threshold. The result is reminiscent of the multicolored images produced by the red-and-white system. The demonstration explicitly confirms our early proposition that the lightness information collected at two wave bands by separate receptor systems is not averaged, point by point and area by area, but is kept distinct and is compared. We know that the rod system does not produce a colored image when the image is seen by itself, and we know that the long-wave light alone cannot produce an image with a variety of colors. The combination, however, gives rise to a wide variety of colors, namely reds, yellows, browns, blue-greens, grays and blacks.

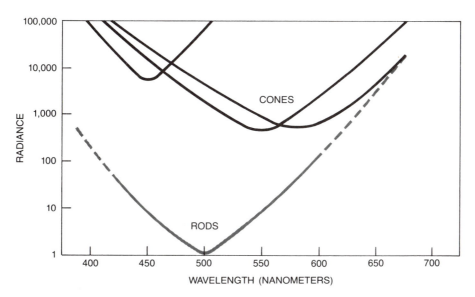

Figure 3.4 THRESHOLD RESPONSES OF RETINAL RE-CEPTORS vary by large factors. The hypersensitive rod system provides vision at radiance levels about 1,000 times weaker than the light levels needed to activate the cone systems. It has been shown in author's laboratory that multicolored scenes exhibit nearly their normal range of colors when they are viewed at light levels so adjusted that only rod system and one cone system, the long-wave system, are responding.

What, then, accounts for the color? The emergence of variegated colors can be ascribed to a process operating somewhere along the visual pathway that compares the lightnesses of the separate images on two wave bands, provided by the two independent retinex systems. The two-receptor experiment makes it plausible that when three independent images constituting the lightnesses of the short-, middle- and long-wave sets of receptors are associated to give a full-colored image, it is the comparison of the respective lightnesses, region by region, that determines the color of each region. The reason the color at any point in an image is essentially independent of the ratio of the three fluxes on three wave bands is that color depends only on the lightness in each wave band and lightness is independent of flux.

As we have seen, the spectral sensitivities of the visual pigments overlap broadly. If we illuminated a scene with the entire range of wavelengths to which a single visual pigment is sensitive, we would see a large variety of colors because more than one retinex system would respond. With the help of filters and appropriate film emulsions, however, we can isolate the lightnesses that would ordinarily be incorporated into the sensation of color. We call black-and-white photographs made for this purpose retinex records.

The photographic technique, making use of silver emulsions, performs two functions. First, the system provides spectral sensitivities that are the same as those of the visual pigments. Second, it generates black-and-white pictures for a human observer to examine. It is the human visual system that converts the photographic pattern deposited in silver into lightness. Ideally we should like our observer to examine the black-and-white pattern with only one set of cones, reporting the lightnesses appropriate to that set. At any point in the black-and-white pattern, however, the reflectance is essentially the same throughout the visible spectrum. Therefore with a black-and-white photograph we stimulate all the receptors with the same information, that is, with the energies that would be absorbed by a single visual pigment. If we assume that all the retinex systems process information in an identical manner, we can propose that sending this identical information to several sets of receptors is the same as sending it to only one receptor, thereby enabling us to see what the image would look like if it were possible to isolate it.

In Figure 3.2, the reader will see three black-and-white pictures taken through retinex filters that simulate the response of the three cone pigments. The strawberries and radishes, for example, are light on the long-wave record, darker on the middle-wave record and darkest on the short-wave record. Although the orange and lemon are about as dark as the strawberries and radishes on the short-wave record, they are nearly as light on the middle-wave record as they are on the long-wave record. On the printed page the distinctions are subtle. To the eye viewing an actual full-color scene the subtle distinctions provide all the information needed to distinguish countless shades and tints of every color.

After the three lightnesses of an area have been determined by the three retinex systems no further information is necessary to characterize the color of any object in the field of view. Any specific color is a report on a trio of three specific lightnesses. For each trio of lightnesses there is a specific and unique color.

The limitations of color photography make it impossible to show the reader the demonstrations readily accomplished in our laboratory, which dramatically reveal the independence of perceived color from the flux reaching the eye. What the reader would see would be two boards four and a half feet square identically covered with about 100 pieces of paper of various colors and shapes. In order to minimize the role of specular reflectance the papers have matte surfaces and, except for black, have a minimum reflectance of at least 10 percent for any part of the visible spectrum. In these displays, which we call "color Mondrians" (after the Dutch painter to whose work they bear a certain resemblance), the papers are arranged so that each one is surrounded by at least five or six others of different colors (see Figure 3.5).

Each of the identical Mondrians is illuminated by its own set of three projectors equipped with sharply cutting band-pass filters (not retinex filters): one at 670 nanometers embracing a band of long waves, one at 540 nanometers embracing a band of middle waves and one at 450 nanometers embracing a band of short waves. The amount of light from each illuminating projector is controlled by a separate variable transformer. In addition the illuminating projectors have synchronized solenoid-activated shutters to control the duration of illumination. There is a telescopic photometer that can be precisely aimed at any region of either Mondrian to

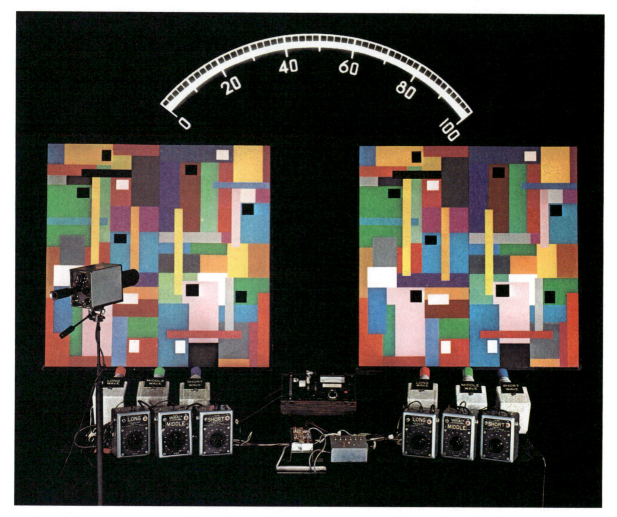

Figure 3.5 "COLOR MONDRIAN' EXPERIMENT employs two identical displays of sheets of colored paper with a matte finish mounted on boards. Each "Mondrian" is illuminated with its own set of three projector illuminators equipped with band-pass filters and independent brightness controls. A telescopic photometer can be pointed at any area to measure the flux, one wave band at a time. In a typical experiment the illuminators can be adjusted so that the white area in the Mondrian at the left and the green area (or some other area) in the Mondrian at the right are both sending the same triplet of radiant energies to the eye. Under actual viewing conditions, white area continues to look white and green area continues to look green even though the eye is receiving the same flux triplet from both areas.

measure the amount of radiation reflected from any point and therefore the amount of flux reaching the eye. The output of the photometer is projected on a scale above the Mondrian, where it can be seen by those taking part in the demonstration.

The demonstration begins with the three illuminating projectors turned on the Mondrian on the left; the Mondrian on the right remains dark. The variable transformers are set so that the entire array of papers in the left Mondrian are deeply colored and at the same time the whites are good whites. This setting is not critical. Then, using one projector at a time and hence only one wave band at a time, we measure with the telescopic photometer the energy reaching the eye from some particular area, say a white rectangle. The readings from the white area (in milliwatts per steradian per square meter) are 65 units of long-wave light, 30 units of middle-wave light and five units of short-wave light. We have now established the three energies associated with that sensation of white.

We turn off the three projectors illuminating the color Mondrian on the left. On the right we turn on only the long-wave projector. We select a different area of unknown color and adjust the long-wave light until the long-wave energy coming to the eye from the selected area is the same as the long-wave energy that a moment ago came from the white paper in the Mondrian on the left, 65 units. We turn off the long-wave projector and separately adjust the transformers controlling the middle- and short-wave projectors, one after the other, so that the energies sent to the eye from the selected area are also the same as those that came from the white area on the left. We have not yet turned on all three light sources simultaneously, but we know that when we do so, the triplet of energies reaching the eye from the selected area of still unknown color will be identical with the triplet that had previously produced the sensation white.

When we turn on the three illuminants, we discover that the area in the Mondrian on the right is green. We now illuminate the Mondrian on the left with its illuminants at their original settings so that both Mondrians can be viewed simultaneously. The white area on the left continues to look white and

the green area on the right continues to look green, yet both are sending to the eye the same triplet of energies: 65, 30 and five in the chosen units (see Figure 3.6).

We turn off the illuminants for both Mondrians and select some other area in the left Mondrian and sequentially adjust the energies reaching the eye from it so that they are the same as the energies that originally gave rise to the sensation of white and also gave rise to the sensation of green in the right Mondrian. When we turn on all three projectors illuminating the left Mondrian, we see that this time the selected area is yellow. The triplet of energies reaching our eye is the same one that had previously produced the sensations of white and green. Again, if we wish, the yellow and green can be viewed simultaneously, with yellow on the left and green on the right.

We can continue the demonstration with other areas such as blue, gray, red and so on. It is dramatically demonstrated that the sensation of color is not related to the product of reflectance times illumination, namely energy, although that product appears to be the only information reaching the eye from the various areas in the Mondrians.

In order to demonstrate that the color sensations in these experiments do not involve extensive chromatic adaptation of retinal pigments the projectors are equipped with synchronized shutters so that the Mondrians can be viewed in a brief flash, a tenth of

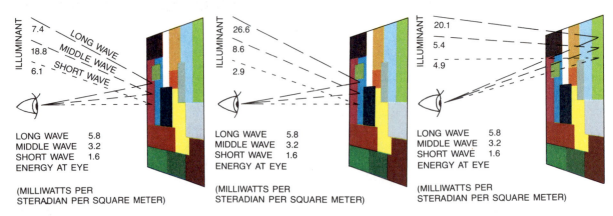

ILLUMINANT 7.4 LONG WAVE 18.8 MIDDLE WAVE 6.1 SHORT WAVE

LONG WAVE 5.8
MIDDLE WAVE 3.2
SHORT WAVE 1.6
ENERGY AT EYE

(MILLIWATTS PER STERADIAN PER SQUARE METER)

ILLUMINANT 26.6 8.6 2.9

LONG WAVE 5.8
MIDDLE WAVE 3.2
SHORT WAVE 1.6
ENERGY AT EYE

(MILLIWATTS PER STERADIAN PER SQUARE METER)

ILLUMINANT 20.1 5.4 4.9

LONG WAVE 5.8
MIDDLE WAVE 3.2
SHORT WAVE 1.6
ENERGY AT EYE

(MILLIWATTS PER STERADIAN PER SQUARE METER)

Figure 3.6 IDENTICAL ENERGY FLUXES AT THE EYE provide different color sensations in the Mondrian experiments. In this example, with the illuminants from the long-wave, middle-wave and short-wave illuminators adjusted as indicated, an area that looks red continues to look red (*left*), an area that looks blue continues to look blue (*middle*) and an area that looks green continues to look green (*right*), even though all three are sending to the eye the same triplet of long-, middle- and short-wave energies. The same triplet can be made to come from any other area: if the area is white, it remains white; if the area is gray, it remains gray; if it is yellow, it remains yellow, and so on.

a second or less in duration. Regardless of the brevity of observation the results of the demonstrations are not altered. Thus one can say that neither chromatic adaptation nor eye motion is involved in producing the observed colors. Finally, the very essence of the design of the color Mondrian is to obviate the significance of the shape and size of surrounding areas, of the familiarity of objects and of the memory of color. Curiously, from time to time there is a casual attempt to adduce what is called color constancy as an explanation of these demonstrations. Clearly color constancy is only a compact designation of the remarkable competence that is the subject of this article.

The mystery is how we can all agree with precision on the colors we see when there is no obvious physical quantity at a point that will enable us to specify the color or an object. Indeed, one can say the stimulus for the color of a point in an area is not the radiation from that point. The task of psychophysics is to find the nature of the stimulus for that color.

Here let us remember that what the eye does unfailingly well is to discover lightness values independent of flux. We say this to be true for a single receptor system, the rod system, operating alone and for the three cone systems operating collectively when they viewed an array of white, gray and black papers. Let us now illuminate the colored Mondrian array with light from just one of the three projectors, say the projector supplying long-wave light, and observe the effect of increasing and decreasing the flux by a large factor. We observe that the various areas maintain a constant rank order of lightness. If, however, we switch the illumination to a different wave band, say the middle wave band, the lightnesses of many of the areas will change; many of the 100 or so areas will occupy a different rank order from lightest to darkest. Under the short-wave-band illuminant there will be yet a third rank order. Specifically, a red paper will be seen as being light in the long-wave light, darker in middle-wave light and very dark in short-wave light. A blue paper, on the other hand, will be light in short-wave light and very dark in both middle- and long-wave light. Papers of other colors will exhibit different triplets of lightnesses. When we conducted such experiments nearly 20 years ago, we were led inevitably to the conclusion that the triplets of lightnesses, area by area, provided the set of constancies we needed to serve as the stimuli for color, independent of flux.

It is evident that the lightnesses exhibited by a given piece of colored paper under illuminants of three different wave bands is related to the amount of energy the paper reflects to the eye at different wavelengths. Let us now examine, by means of a particular experiment, how such reflectances can be related step by step to perceived lightnesses and how, in the process, the radiant flux that reaches the eye—the ultimate source of knowledge about lightness—finally becomes irrelevant to the sensation of color.

In our laboratory McCann, Suzanne P. McKee and Thomas H. Taylor made a systematic study of observers' responses to a simplified color Mondrian with areas of 17 different colors. They asked the observers to match the 17 areas one at a time under different illuminants with colored squares of paper that had been selected from a standard color-reference book, *The Munsell Book of Color*, and that were viewed under a constant "white" illumination.

The illuminants on the Mondrian were adjusted in five separate matching experiments so that five different areas (gray, red, yellow, blue and green) sent to the eye an identical triplet of radiances. The observer began by selecting a matching Munsell "chip" for each of the 17 areas in the Mondrian when the gray area in the Mondrian sent a particular triplet of energies to the eye. Another set of 17 matching Munsell chips was selected when the same triplet was later sent to the eye by a red area in the Mondrian, and the same was done for yellow, blue and green areas under illuminants that supplied the same triplet of energies.

Figures 3.7, 3.8, 3.9 and 3.10 show the details of the experiment and the five different Munsell colors the observers selected to match the five areas when each area sent to the eye precisely the same triplet of energies. In spite of the constancy of the energy reaching one eye from the Mondrian, each observer, using the other eye, selected Munsell chips that were gray, red, yellow, blue and green.

The constant illumination used in viewing the Munsell book was a triplet of illuminants at three wavelengths that observers judged to produce the "best" white. The actual triplet of wavelengths reaching the eye from the whitest paper in the Munsell book was 11.5 units of long-wave light, 7.8 units of middle-wave light and 3.3 units of short-wave light. The illuminants supplied energy in narrow bands with peaks at 630 nanometers, 530 nanometers and 450 nanometers. A similar triplet of

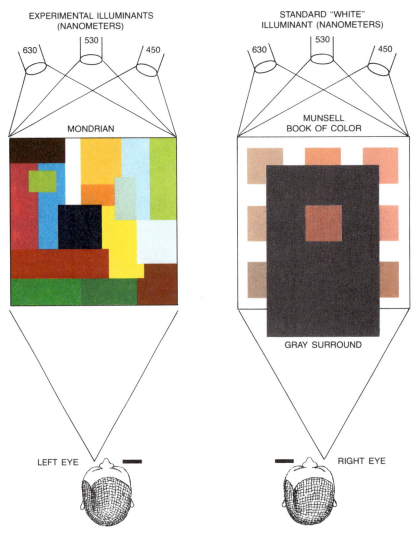

Figure 3.7 COLOR-MATCHING EXPERIMENT uses a simplified Mondrian (*left*) and standard color reference "chips" (*right*). The Mondrian is illuminated with three narrow-band light sources (see text), the ratio of which is such that the energies reflected to the eye from any area equals those that previously reached the eye from some other area. In this experiment different color areas were selected in sequence to send the same energies to the eye, and for each one the observer selected the chip that came closest to matching it. The chips were illuminated with a constant spectral mixture of three narrow-band lights so that the white chip appeared the "best white." One eye was used for viewing the Mondrian and the other for viewing chips. The chip was always surrounded by the same gray paper.

narrow-band illuminants were mixed in various proportions to illuminate the Mondrian.

At this point the reader might ask: Would not a single gray area exhibit a pronounced change in color if the surrounding papers had reflected light of widely differing spectral composition? Could these changes in color account for the results of the Mon-

drian experiments? The answer to the questions is that no manipulation of surrounding papers in the Mondrian is capable of making the gray paper match the red, yellow, blue, and green Munsell papers selected by the observers in the Mondrian experiment.

McCann, John A. Hall and I have examined the

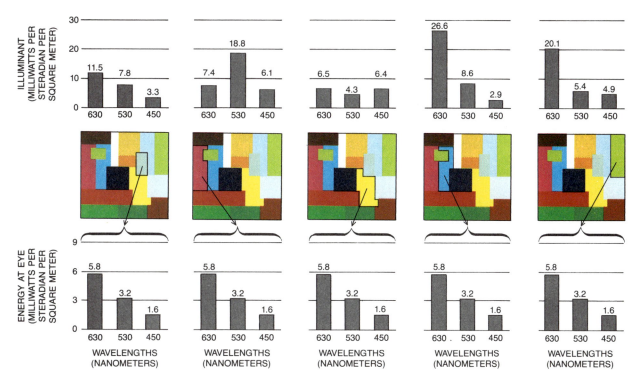

Figure 3.8 PROPORTIONS OF NARROW-BAND ILLU-MINANTS used to light the simplified Mondrian in the Munsell-chip matching experiments were adjusted as is shown by the bars at the top of this illustration so that five different areas of the Mondrian (*indicated by arrows*) sent to the observer's eye in successive matching trials the same triplet of energies: 5.8 flux units of long-wave light, 3.2 flux units of middle-wave light and 1.6 flux units of short-wave light. Figure 3.9 shows the Munsell chips that were selected in the constant illuminant to match the five Mondrian areas (gray, red, yellow, blue and green) that had sent to the eye exactly the same triplet of energies.

matter further by repeating the Mondrian-Munsell experiment in various ways so that the average spectral composition of the light reaching the eye from the Mondrian and its surround remains the same regardless of the spectral composition of the light needed to establish a constant triplet from area to area. We have done this in one case by surrounding the entire Mondrian with brightly colored papers selected in such a way that they exactly offset the average mixture of wave bands from the Mondrian itself and, more dramatically, by cutting the 17 areas of the Mondrian apart and placing them well separated on the backgrounds of offsetting color. Neither arrangement has any significant effect on the Munsell chips chosen to match the various areas of the Mondrian.

L et us return, then, to the search for the stimulus that guides us so accurately to the correct iden-

tification of colors. If it is not a flux of radiant energy at the eye from each point in the field of view, what are the physical correlates of the lightnesses of objects on three separate wave bands, corresponding to the spectral sensitivities of the cone pigments? Can such a precise physical correlate of lightness be demonstrated?

McCann, McKee and Taylor next measured the radiance, or energy at the eye, of the various Mondrian areas and of the matching Munsell chips by using a photomultiplier in conjunction with a version of the retinex filters. Since the retinex-photomultiplier combination integrates the flux of radiant energy over a broad band of wavelengths, the instrument provides a value we call integrated radiance. McCann and his colleagues then obtained the integrated radiances from a large sheet of white paper placed under each of the experimental illuminants that had been used to light the Mondrian in the chip-matching experiments. If the integrated radiance from a Mondrian area is used as the numerator in a fraction and the integrated radiance from the white paper is used as the denominator, one obtains a value for integrated reflectance, which can be expressed as a percent.

The integrated reflectances for the various Munsell chips are determined in the same manner under the constant "white" illumination. This amounts to measuring the percentage of reflectance using detectors with the same spectral sensitivity as the visual pigments. The results show that the Munsell chip chosen by the eye to match a given Mondrian area will have approximately the same three integrated reflectances as the area. For example, the blue area in the Mondrian has a triplet of integrated reflectances (long, middle- and short-wave) of 27.3, 35.9 and 60.7 percent. The comparable values for

Figure 3.10 FURTHER ANALYSIS OF MATCHING EXPERIMENT begins to identify the basis on which the visual system makes the color match between the Mondrian area and the Munsell chip without regard to the flux each member of the pair sends to the eye. The efficiency with which a given area in the Mondrian reflects light in each of the three wave bands (*first column*) multiplied by the amount of energy striking that area in each of the wave bands (*second column*) yields the energy triplet that reaches the eye (*third column*). The three columns at the right contain comparable data for the Munsell chips selected as a match for the Mondrian areas.

the matched Munsell chip are 34.6, 38.5 and 57.1 percent (see Figure 3.11).

Finally, the integrated reflectances are "scaled" so that their equal spacing is consistent with the equal spacing of lightness sensations. The curve for this transformation is shown in Figure 3.12. Using this

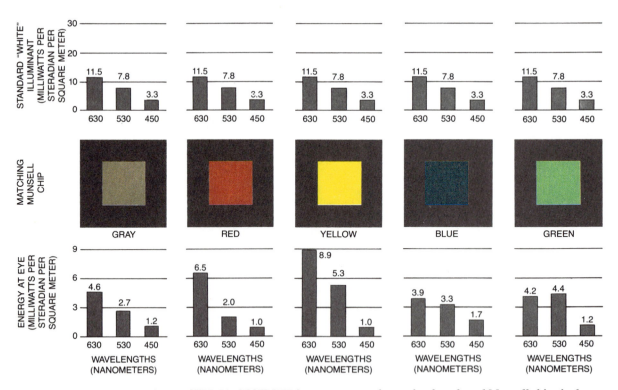

Figure 3.9 MUNSELL CHIPS SELECTED BY OBSERVERS to match the five Mondrian areas that had sent identical triplets of energy to the eye are reproduced. The Munsell book was illuminated with a constant spectral mixture of narrow-band illuminants (*bars at top*) and the chips were viewed within a constant gray surround. The energy that was sent to the eye by the selected Munsell chips is shown by the bars at the bottom of the illustration. It is evident that the match between the Mondrian areas and the Munsell chips is not made on the basis of the flux of radiant energy at the eye of the observer. What does cause the two areas to match is described in the illustrations that follow.

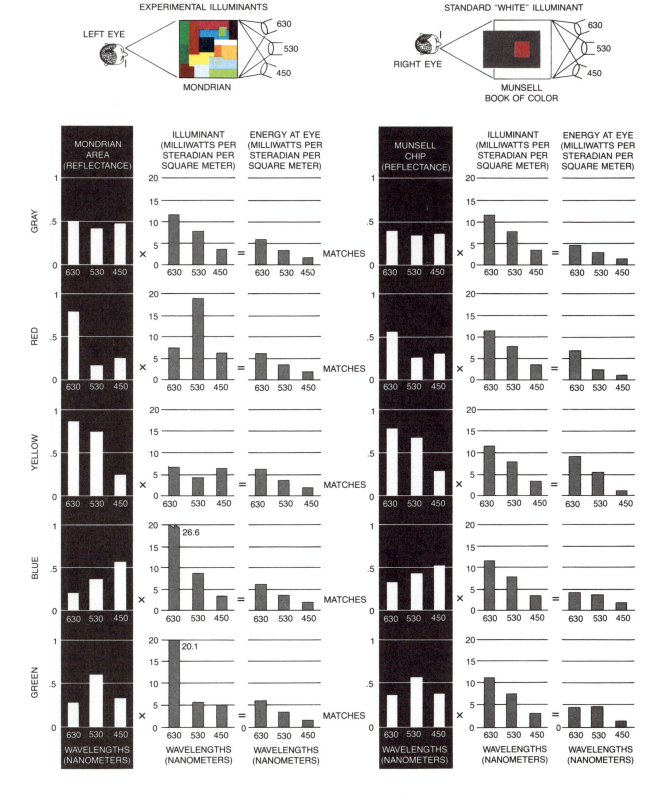

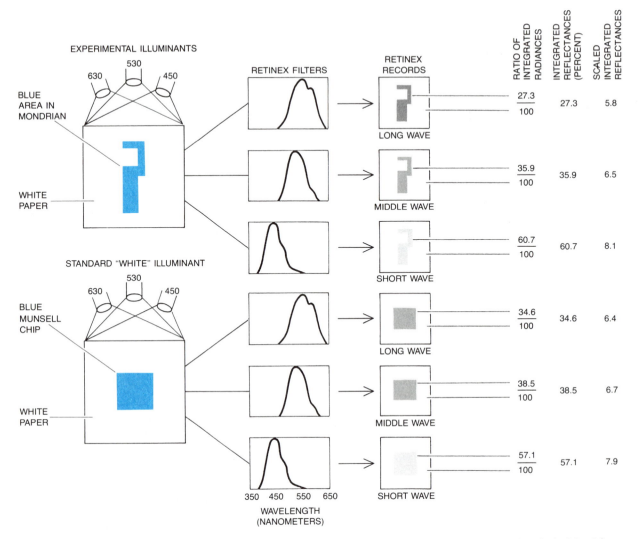

Figure 3.11 ROLE OF REFLECTANCE and its psychophysical correlate, lightness, in guiding the eye to match Munsell chips with Mondrian areas was examined with the help of retinex filter-photomultiplier combinations that match the spectral sensitivity of the cone pigments. Under each combination of illuminants (*top*) the integrated radiance, or flux, in each retinex wave band of a Mondrian area was compared with the integrated radiance of a sheet of white paper. The ratio of integrated radiances yields the integrated reflectance of the Mondrian area, expressed here in percent. For the matching Munsell chip a set of ratios was similarly determined (*bottom*).

curve, we see that the blue area in the Mondrian has a triplet of scaled integrated reflectances of 5.8, 6.5 and 8.1, whereas the corresponding values for the matching Munsell chip are 6.4, 6.7 and 7.9. If we study the five areas that successively sent identical triplets of energies to the eye and compare their scaled integrated reflectances with those of their matching Munsell chips, we find that all the values are in excellent agreement. In others words, in the triplets of integrated reflectances we have identified a highly accurate physical correlate of color sensations. The data fall along the 45-degree line that describes the locus of perfect correlation (see Figure 3.13).

We have sought a physical correlate for lightness, and we have found that the scaled integrated reflec-

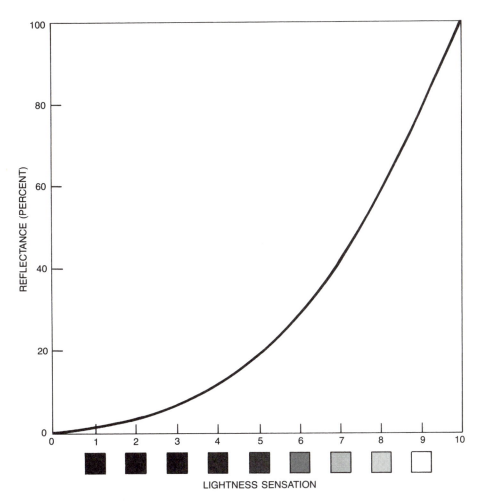

Figure 3.12 SENSATION OF LIGHTNESS is plotted on an equal-interval scale. Observers are shown a sheet of white paper (9) and a sheet of black paper (1) and are then asked to choose a sheet of paper whose shade of gray lies halfway between the two. The selection is the gray labeled 5. Similar selections are made to determine the locations of midpoints between 1 and 5 and between 5 and 9 and so on until the equal-interval scale is filled. The end values 0 and 10 are extrapolations. The curve, plotted by measuring the reflectances of the various selected papers, makes it possible to convert values of integrated reflectance into values of scaled integrated reflectance, as given in the far right column of Figure 3.11.

tances of the five areas that sent identical triplets of fluxes to our eyes are the same as those of the matching Munsell chip. This correlation enables us to use scaled integrated reflectances as a measured lightness equivalent. The problem now shifts to one of how the eye derives the lightness that corresponds to the reflectances of objects in each wave band.

It is one thing to measure a triplet of lightness equivalents using a retinex filter coupled to a photo-

multiplier; it is quite another for the eye to determine lightnesses in the unevenly lighted world without reference sheets of white paper. I described above the ability of an isolated receptor system—the hypersensitive system of rod vision—to classify objects correctly according to their inherent reflectivity regardless of whether the objects happened to be in a brightly or a dimly lighted region of visual space. The ability of one receptor system to work in this way makes it plausible that the other three

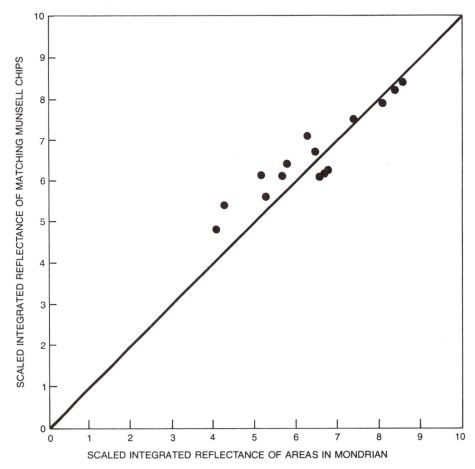

Figure 3.13 AGREEMENT IN SCALED INTEGRATED REFLECTANCES between Mondrian areas and Munsell chips is summarized for all three wave-band systems. The scaled integrated reflectances of five Mondrian areas and matching chips were determined as in Figure 3.11. This graph plots triplets of scaled integrated reflectances of five Mondrian areas that sent identical fluxes to the eye against scaled integrated reflectances of matched Munsell chips. The dots collectively represent correspondence for all three retinex wave bands; any particular dot denotes the degree of correspondence on one retinex wave band between a Mondrian area and a Munsell chip.

systems of normal daytime vision possess the same ability, each system viewing the world through a broad but restricted region of the spectrum, the regions we duplicate with retinex filters. Each system forms a separate lightness image of the world. The images are not mixed but compared. The comparison of lightnesses at each area gives rise to the range of sensations we know as color.

How could the biological system generate a hierarchy and spacing of lightness values given only the flux from each point in a scene and knowing nothing about the pattern of illumination and nothing about the reflectances of objects? The scheme I am about to describe is the most general we have found that surmounts these limitations; its physiological embodiment could take many forms.

Let me begin by pointing out the significance of edges in defining objects or areas in a scene. If a sheet of white paper is lighted strongly from one side, we see no discontinuity in color from one side to the other. Let us now imagine two light detectors positioned to measure the luminance from two different places on the paper. If the illumination is nonuniform, the luminances of the two places will of course be different. As the two detectors are moved closer together the luminances approach the same value and ratio of the two outputs approaches unity. If, however, the two detectors bridge the boundary between two areas that differ abruptly in reflectance, such as would be the case with even a pale gray square on the white paper, the ratio of the outputs of the two detectors will approach the ratio of the two reflectances [The ratio is subjected to a threshold test: any ratio to be regarded as a change must vary from unity by more than some small threshold amount, plus or minus .003 in the computer program]. Thus the single procedure of taking the ratio between two adjacent points can both detect an edge and eliminate the effect of nonuniform illumination. If we process the entire image in terms of the ratios of luminances at closely adjacent points, we can generate dimensionless numbers that are independent of the illumination. These numbers give the ratio of reflectances at the edge between adjacent areas; the reflectances themselves are not yet ascertained.

In order to determine reflectances we need to relate all these ratios of reflectances in the field of view. Given the ratio of luminances at the edge between a first area and a second one, we multiply it by the ratio of luminances at the edge between the second area and a third. This product of ratios approaches the ratio of reflectances between the first and third areas, regardless of the distribution of illumination. Similarly, we can obtain the ratio of reflectances of any two areas in an image, however remote they are from each other, by multiplying the ratios of all the boundaries between the starting area and the remote area. We can also establish the ratio of the reflectance of any area on the path by tapping off the sequential product reached at that area (see Figures 3.14 and 3.15).

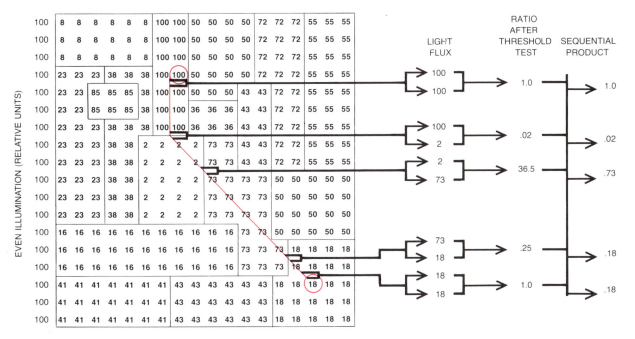

Figure 3.14 SCHEME FOR EYE'S METHOD of discovering lightness in complex images is depicted here and in Figure 3.15. The numbers inside the schematic Mondrian represent the long-wave integrated radiances coming from each area of a display that is evenly lighted. The long-wave retinex system independently "measures" the long-wave integrated radiance, point by point, as if along an arbitrary pathway (*color*). The flux at each successive closely spaced pair of points is converted into a ratio. If the ratio does not vary from unity by some threshold amount, it is regarded as being "unchanged" and is set to equal unity. A second threshold-tested ratio along the same pathway is multiplied by the first ratio to give a sequential product that is both the model's response for that point and the signal sent along to be multiplied by the next ratio. When the path crosses an edge between two lightnesses, there is a sharp change in the threshold-tested ratio and hence a similar change in the sequential product.

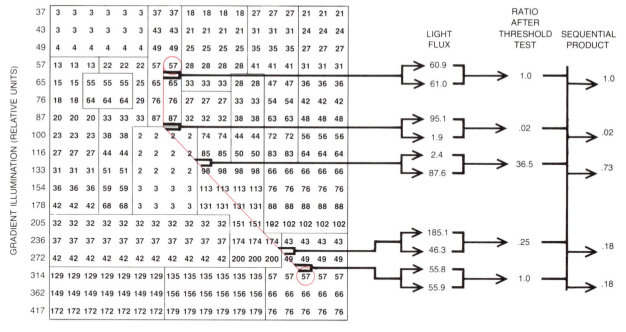

Figure 3.15 MORE REALISTIC CASE OF GRADED ILLU-MINATION is handled equally well by the sequential-product method to arrive at the same reflectance value of .18 for the brown area at the end of the path, even though here the long-wave retinex system receives as much flux from the middle of the brown area (57) as it does from the middle of the white area (57). (The white and brown areas are shown in color in Figures 3.6, 3.7 and 3.8.) The scheme hence provides a means for arriving at computed reflectance independent of flux and without resort to white cards as standards. Precise values of light flux along pathway in this diagram were derived from a computer program that works with 75 values between every two values printed within Mondrian.

We are now coming close to the answer to the question: How can the eye ascertain the reflectance of an area without in effect placing a comparison standard next to the area? The sequential product can be used as a substitute for the placement of two areas adjacent to each other, thus defining a photometric operation feasible for the eye.

The remaining task is to suggest how the eye can discover the area of highest reflectance in the field of view and then decide whether that area is actually white or some other color. In the model we have proposed, sequential products are computed along many arbitrary pathways that wander through the two-dimensional array of energies on the model's "retina." Since the pathways can begin anywhere, not just in regions of the highest reflectance, the first value in any sequence is arbitrarily assumed to be 100 percent. [Thus, in Figure 3.14, the path is started in the white area, where the flux of radiant energy is 100. By the time the path reaches the brown area at the lower right, the product is .18. (The corresponding colored areas are shown in Figures 3.6, 3.7 and 3.8.) The retinex system has thus determined that the brown area reflects 18 percent as much long-wave energy as the white area. Any other path ending in the brown area would yield the same result as long as it had been through the white area. By averaging the responses for each area, as computed by many arbitrary paths, the long-wave retinex system arrives at a single reflectance value for each area, which designates perceived lightness. Middle- and short-wave retinex systems compute their own sets of lightness values. Comparison of triplet of lightnesses for each area provides sensation of color.] Because of this deliberately adopted fiction the sequential product becomes greater than unity whenever the path reaches an area whose reflectance is higher than that of the starting area.

The attainment of a sequential product greater than unity indicates that the sequence should be started afresh with the new area of high reflectance taken as being 100 percent. This procedure is the heart of the technique for finding the highest reflectance in the path. After the path reaches the highest reflectance in the scene, each of the sequential products computed thereafter becomes a fraction of the highest value. A satisfactory computer program has been designed to study the number of paths, their lengths and convolutions, the threshold values for recognizing edges and, perhaps most important, how to utilize all the pathways starting in all areas.

The biological counterpart of this program is performed in undetermined parts of the pathway between the retina and the cortex. The process that corresponds to computing sequential products does not involve the averaging of areas or the averaging of flux. It does, however, call for an arithmetic that extends over the entire visual field. Furthermore, since the relevant phenomena are seen in a brief pulse of light, all the computations and conclusions about lightness must be carried out in a fraction of a second without dependence on eye movement. With a single pulse, eye movement, by definition, is not necessary. With continuous illumination the normal quick motions of the eye probably serve to maintain the freshness of the process.

With our computer model we can obtain a triplet of lightnesses for each area in the color Mondrian that corresponds closely to the lightnesses one would measure with a combined retinex filter and photomultiplier. The color corresponding to any given triplet can be visualized with the aid of the color "solid" we have built, in which the Munsell colors are located in three dimensions in "lightness-color space" according to their lightness values measured in three wave bands through retinex filters. [Each plane in Figure 3.16 is the locus of colors possible with a constant short-wave lightness. For example, the fifth plane from the bottom shows the variety of color sensations from all possible long- and middle-wave lightness values, when those values are combined with a short-wave lightness of 5. The colored squares are samples taken from *The Munsell Book of Color*. In general the blank areas on each plane represent regions where colors, if they were produced at all, could be produced only by fluorescent dyes.]

In normal images the sensation of white light will be generated by any area that is placed at the top of the lightness scale by all three retinex systems. On the other hand, an area that stands at the top of only two of the three lightness scales will be seen as some other color. Hence an area that is at the top of

the lightness scale in the long- and middle-wave systems but is surpassed in lightness by some other area in the short-wave system will be seen not as white but as yellow. A similar intercomparison of triplets of lightnesses at the same place within each scene provides the sensation of color, area by area, in spite of unpredictable variations in illumination.

If one looks at black-and-white photographs taken through retinex filters, one sees a dramatic difference in lightness for most objects between the photograph representing the short-wave system and either of the photographs representing the other two systems. And yet it is the comparatively small differences between the long-wave and the middle-wave lightnesses that are responsible for the experience of vivid reds and greens.

Such reliable and sensitive responsiveness to small lightness differences provides the basis for the colors seen under anomalous conditions far removed from those the eye has evolved to see. Two examples of interest are the color of a spot of light in a total surrounding area devoid of light and the spectrum of colors produced by a prism.

One can readily measure the flux at the eye from a spot of light in a void. By changing the flux it is possible to estimate the corresponding change in perceived lightness. What one finds is that the estimated lightness changes only slowly with enormous changes in flux. For example, decreasing the flux by a very large amount will be seen as a very small reduction in lightness. If the spot of light is composed of a narrow band of long wavelength, say 600 nanometers, one can expect all three cone receptors to absorb the radiation in some degree, but significantly more radiation will be absorbed by the long-wave cones than by the other two kinds. [In arbitrary units the long-wave pigment might absorb 80 units, the middle-wave pigment 20 units and the short-wave pigment a few tenths of a unit at most.] When the three values are read on a scale of perceived lightness, the three lightnesses are 9 on the long-wave system, 8.5 on the middle-wave system and 7.5 on the short-wave system (see Figure 3.17). This combination of lightnesses is seen as a light reddish orange, a color not commonly perceived under ordinary conditions unless the surfaces are fluorescent. The spectrum, a strikingly anomalous display, can be regarded as a series of three laterally displaced continuous gradients involving both the properties of spots and the properties of areas. From these properties it is possible to predict the colors of the spectrum, whereas it is not possible, as we have

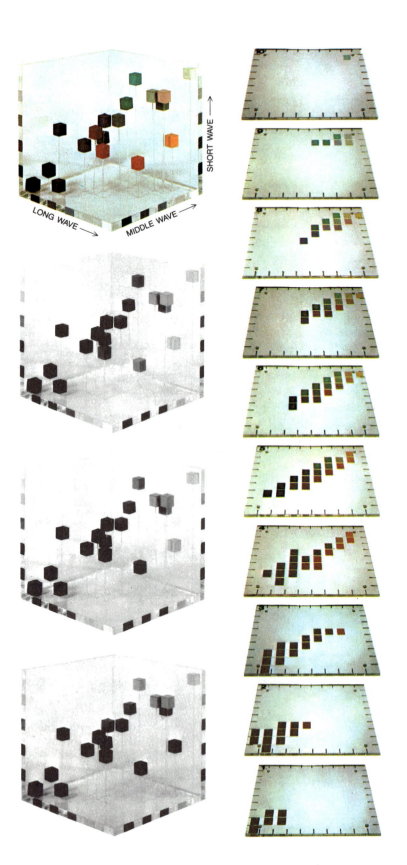

Figure 3.16 COLOR "SOLID" locates all perceivable colors, including white and black. The position of a color in this three-dimensional space is determined by the triplet of lightness computed by the eye for each area. The color photograph at the top left shows the location of representative colors throughout the space. The direction of increasing lightness along each axis is shown by the arrows. The three black-and-white photographs of the color solid were taken with retinex filter-film combinations. They show the lightness values of the representative colors as they would be perceived separately by the eye's long-wave (top), middle-wave (middle) and short-wave (bottom) visual pigments. The set of 10 color pictures at the right represents horizontal planes cut through the three-dimensional color space.

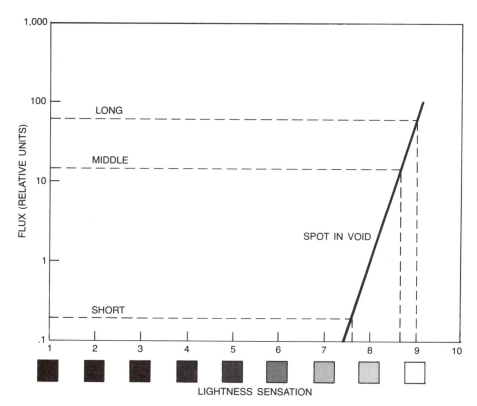

Figure 3.17 SPOT OF LIGHT IN A VOID, that is, a single spot of narrow-band light viewed in an otherwise totally dark environment, has a color that would seem to depend solely on its wavelength. The color can also be explained, however, by the retinex theory in terms of lightness as perceived by the eye's three receptor systems. Psychophysical measurements show that when the eye is presented with a spot of light in a void, the perceived lightness is changed only slightly by very large changes in flux, as is indicated by the straight line.

seen, to attribute a specific spectral composition to the radiance from a colored area in everyday life.

Perhaps the first observation pointedly relevant to the mechanism of color formation in images is not Newton's spectrum but the phenomenon of colored shadows, described in 1672 by Otto von Guericke. "This is how it happens," he wrote, "that in the early morning twilight a clear blue shadow can be produced upon a white piece of paper [by holding] a finger or other object . . . between a lighted candle and the paper beneath." This important experiment, we now know, depicts an elementary example of generating three different lightnesses on the three receptor systems. A diagram of this experiment with long-wave ("red") light and white light appears in Figure 3.18. Here the color of the shadow is blue-green. [In the analysis at the right in Figure 3.18 it is assumed that one projector

sends white light to the screen. The other projector, equipped with a red filter, sends only long wavelengths to the screen. Assume that the white light contributes 100 arbitrary units of flux to each of the short-, middle- and long-wave receptors. The long-wave flux is absorbed by the three receptor systems in different proportions: 100 units are absorbed by the long-wave system, 50 by the middle-wave system and five by the short-wave system. (A small amount of scattered long-wave light also appears in the shadow.) The third column of boxes shows the combined amounts of flux from both sources absorbed by each receptor system. The fractions represent the ratio at edges of the flux from within the shadow divided by the flux from outside. The fourth column shows the lightness on each receptor system. The lightness of the lightest place in the scene for each receptor system will be near the top of the lightness scale, being determined by the flux

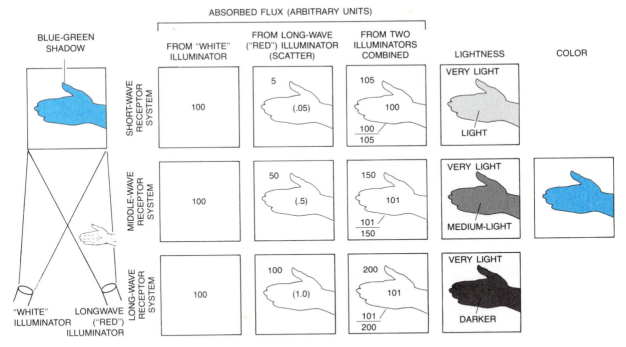

Figure 3.18 BLUE-GREEN COLORED SHADOW is seen when a hand or some other object is placed in the beam of a projector that is sending long-wave ("red") light to a screen while the screen is illuminated by a beam of white light. **The author regards Otto von Guericke's description in 1672 of seeing colored shadows made by candlelight as the first observation pointedly relevant to the mechanism of image and color formation.**

of radiant energy in the same way that a spot has its lightness determined by flux. Triplet of lightnesses within the shadow falls in the region of color space that the eye perceives as being blue-green.] The diagram thus shows that the triplet of lightnesses in the shadow corresponds to the blue-green color one would predict for it from its position in lightness-color space.

One can now understand the red-and-white images of our early work as a procedure that carries the colored shadow to a richly variegated family of colors no longer in shadows but in images. The colors seen in a red-and-white projection can be readily predicted by extending the analysis followed in predicting the color of von Guericke's shadow. To demonstrate this point we reproduce in Figure 3.19 the "red" and "green" separation images used in making a red-and-white multicolored projection. (In this demonstration no attempt is made to reproduce the colors seen in the actual multicolored image.) The red-and-white projection was photographed through long-, middle- and short-wave re-

tinex film-filter combinations. The three images are reproduced below the pair of long- and middle-wave separation images that were superposed to make the red-and-white image. [The long-wave record was projected onto a screen with a long-wave (red) filter in the beam of light. The middle-wave record was projected in superposition onto the same screen in the light of a tungsten-filament lamp.] The significant point is that when the eye views the red-and-white images on the screen with its own retinex system, it is provided with a triplet of lightnesses for each part of the scene that resembles the triplet it would obtain if it viewed the original scene directly. In this important meeting point of the blue-green shadows with the colored images, provided by the red-and-white display, the extended taking and multiplication of ratios determine the lightness of each small area. Finally, all these principles are applied in everyday ternary vision, which creates a distinct lightness image for each of the three sensitive systems and compares them in order to generate color.

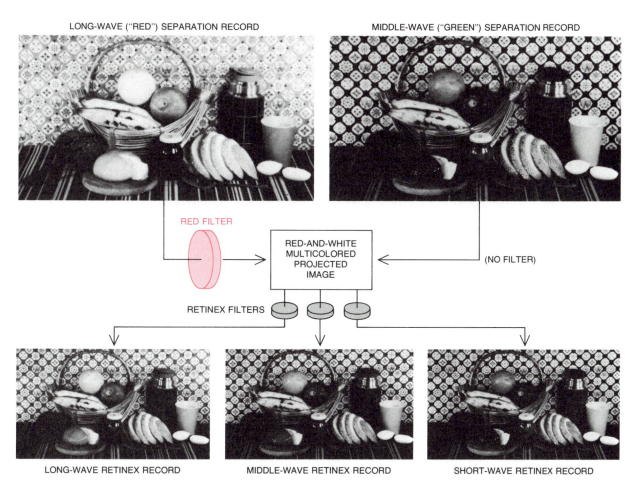

LONG-WAVE ("RED") SEPARATION RECORD

MIDDLE-WAVE ("GREEN") SEPARATION RECORD

RED FILTER

RED-AND-WHITE
MULTICOLORED
PROJECTED
IMAGE

(NO FILTER)

RETINEX FILTERS

LONG-WAVE RETINEX RECORD

MIDDLE-WAVE RETINEX RECORD

SHORT-WAVE RETINEX RECORD

Figure 3.19 RETINEX RECORDS OF RED-AND-WHITE projections show that red-and-white images produce a triplet of lightnesses for each part of the scene consistent with observed color sensations. The two photographs (*top half*) are reproductions of the long-wave (*left*) and middle-wave (*right*) separation records taken of the original still life. The retinex records are reproduced at the bottom: long-wave at the left, middle-wave in the middle and short-wave at the right. The colors seen in red-and-white projections are those one would expect from their triplets of lightnesses. The apple is light on the long record and darker in the middle and short records. The orange is lightest on the long record, intermediate on the middle record and darkest on the short. With one's own retinex systems, one can see a blue cup, a brown straw basket and pale yellow bananas with lightness differences so small as to challenge photoengraving process used to reproduce photographs.

The train of interlocking concepts and experiments started 25 years ago with the observation that the relative energies of the red-and-white projectors can be altered without changing the names of the various colors. This observation negated the simplistic explanation in terms of contrast, fatigue and surround and led to the fundamental concept of independent long- and short-wave image-forming systems that ultimately evolved to the concept of three independent retinex systems and to the Mondrian demonstration. The concept of the percentage of available light on each wave band as a determining variable and the technique of measuring it evolved to the concept that lightnesses maintain an independent rank order on long- and short-wave bands. This measuring technique in turn evolved from a projected black-and-white image to an arrangement of colored papers in the color Mondrian.

The manifest stability and constancy of the lightnesses of all the papers of the Mondrian when a single wave band illuminates it with varying intensity dramatizes the concept that every colored paper has three reflectances on three wave bands and that these reflectances are somehow connected with the biological characteristic: lightnesses.

A black-and-white Mondrian taught that nonuniformity of illumination, size and shape of area and length of edges were basically irrelevant to lightness. What was needed was a far-reaching, edge-reading arithmetic: the sequential product of ratios at edges. For the color Mondrian the ratio at edges was early recognized as requiring a ratio of the integrals of the product at each wavelength of the absorbance of the cone pigment times the reflectance of the colored paper times the illuminants. Separate integrals were taken over the wave bands of the three cone pigments. In a long series of binocular comparison-and-selection observations the quantity satisfying the integral was shown to be impressively well correlated with lightness, particularly after the realization that the scale, or spacing, of the reflectance integral should be made to correspond with the spacing of the biological quantity lightness. This led to the designation "scaled integrated reflectance" as the external partner to which the retinex system relates the internal partner: constructed lightness.

Color can be arranged in the lightness solid with long-, middle-and short-wave axes of lightness. All visible colors reside in this solid independent of flux, each color having a unique position given by the three axial values of lightness. It should be remembered that the reality of color lies in this solid. When the color Mondrian is nonuniformly illuminated, photographed and measured, reflectance in the photograph no longer correlates with the color but the lightness does. The three sets of ratios of integrals at edges and the product of these integrals within a set emerge as the physical determinants in the partnership between the biological system and areas in the external world.

The Perception of Surface Blacks and Whites

What shade of gray a surface appears is related to the perceived distribution of light and shadow, which in turn depends on the perceived spatial relation between the surface and its neighbors.

. . .

Alan L. Gilchrist
March, 1979

The lens of the human eye projects onto the retina a two-dimensional image of the three-dimensional physical world. Partly because the retinal image is two-dimensional most investigators of color perception have assumed that depth perception has nothing to do with the process by which the human visual system determines the color of objects. The experiments I shall describe here invalidate that assumption. I have found that a change in the perceived spatial orientation of a surface can change its perceived color from black to white or from white to black.

Traditional explanations of color perception assign no special role to the central nervous system. Because that system governs depth perception my work assigns it a major role. Traditional investigations have also largely ignored the perception of the intensity and color of the light illuminating surfaces whose colors are under scrutiny. In my work I have tried to rectify this imbalance, and for the sake of simplicity I have dealt mainly with what are called neutral colors: white, black and gray.

When white light, which consists of a balanced mixture of all the colors in the spectrum, strikes a colored surface, the surface reflects one wavelength (one color) more than it does the others. This domi-

nant wavelength corresponds to the physical color of the surface. In general the light that illuminates objects in nature is not white but is an unbalanced mixture of various colors. A colored surface reflects some wavelengths in such a mixture more than others, but now the dominant wavelengths do not correspond to the physical color of the surface. The mixture of wavelengths in the light the surface reflects to the eye depends not only on the physical color of the surface but also on the mixture of wavelengths in the light that illuminates the surface. Therefore the visual system should not be considered an instrument that measures the wavelength and the intensity of reflected light; such measurements would reveal little about surface color. The visual system has the remarkable ability to correctly perceive the physical color of a surface in spite of wide variations in the mixture of wavelengths in the illumination. This is the phenomenon of color constancy.

Neutral surfaces leave unchanged the mixture of wavelengths that illuminates them, but they do alter the intensity of the light. The shades of gray from white to black are all neutral, and so they reflect various degrees of illumination. Surfaces that reflect between about 80 and 90 percent of the illumina-

tion are called white, whereas those that reflect between about 3 and 5 percent are called black. In
short, the lightness, or perceived grayness, of a neutral surface corresponds to its reflectance: the percentage of illumination it reflects. Again, the visual
system has the remarkable ability to determine the
lightness of a neutral surface in spite of wide variations in the intensity of the illumination. Such is the
phenomenon of lightness constancy, which is analogous to the phenomenon of color constancy for
colored surfaces.

A physicist would determine the reflectance of a
surface by comparing the intensity of the reflected light with the intensity of the illumination.
The human visual system also determines reflectance, but it does so by comparing the intensity of
the light reflected from a surface with the intensity
of the light reflected from neighboring surfaces (see
Figure 4.1). For the visual system to make this comparison there must be constant relative displacement between the retinal image and the retina. This
happens naturally because the eye constantly and
involuntarily flicks back and forth in tremors with a
frequency of between 30 and 150 cycles per second.
It has been found that the visual field goes blank in
one to three seconds if the relative displacement is
eliminated by artificially stabilizing the image (using
a special apparatus that causes the image to remain
still on the retina even as the eye moves back and
forth). The eye tremors indicate that the receptor
cells of the retina function only in the presence of a
change of stimulation. Consider what happens to an
individual receptor cell during the tremors (assuming that there are no large voluntary eye movements). A cell in the interior of a patch of homogeneous stimulation within the retinal image receives
no change of stimulation, whereas a cell at the
boundary of a patch does receive such a change.
(See Figure 4.2.)

The relevance of all of this for color vision was
elegantly demonstrated by John Krauskopf of AT&T
Bell Laboratories. He built a display that consisted
of a disk of one color, say green, surrounded by an
annulus, or ring, of another color, say red. He arranged matters so that the green-red boundary between the disk and the annulus was stabilized, that
is, moved in such a way as to follow the tremors. In
this way all displacement between the green-red
boundary and the receptor cells was eliminated. As
a result the retinal boundary disappeared and the
observer simply saw a single large red disk. (See
Figure 4.3.)

The most straightforward interpretation of this
experiment is that the eye sends the brain only information about changes in light across boundaries,
with areas where no change is reported being filled
in by the brain as homogeneous. In Krauskopf's
display, and in the normal viewing of a large red
disk, the eye extracts information from the outer
edge. Since no change is reported within the boundary, the brain treats the interior of the disk as homogeneous. Consider what this implies. Krauskopf's
observers perceived red even in the center of the
display, even though green light was striking the
corresponding region of the retina. Hence if the
color of the light (green) striking the disk region of
the retina had nothing to do with the color (red) that
was perceived there, then by the same token the
color of the light (red) striking the annulus region
might have nothing to do with the color (red) that
was perceived there.

Krauskopf's display suggests that even under natural conditions the perceived color of a surface depends not on the light emanating from the surface
but on the change in the light across the boundary
of the surface. The perceived color of a surface cannot depend solely on the change in the light at the
edge of the surface because such a change is strictly
relative. The change in the light at the edge of a
surface depends as much on the color of the background as it does on the color of the surface.

If perceived color depended only on the change
in the light at the edge of a surface, the surface
would look radically different in color when seen
against different backgrounds. Conversely, two surfaces of radically different color could look the
same. For example, the change in the intensity of
reflected light from a white surface to a middle-gray
background is the same as the change in the intensity from a middle-gray surface to a black background. Of course, white and middle-gray surfaces
would not look the same when they were seen
against these respective backgrounds. Such changes
in background color can result in what are called
contrast effects, but these effects are not nearly
large enough to make the white surface on the middle-gray background look the same as the middle-
gray surface on the black background. It is a remarkable empirical fact that perceived surface color
remains largely constant in spite of changes in the
background, which in turn give rise to changes in
the edge information.

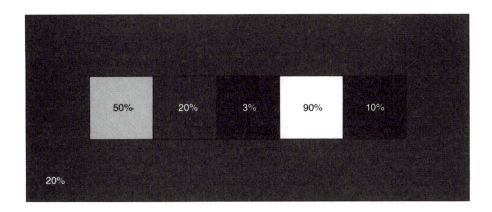

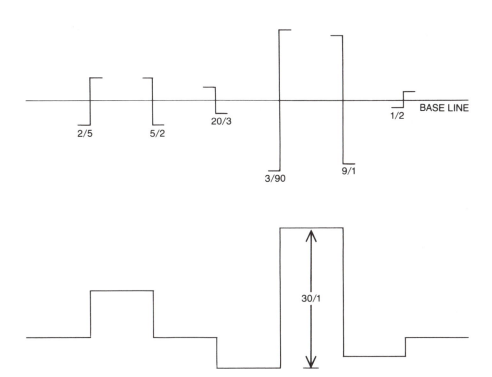

Figure 4.1 REFLECTANCE OF A SURFACE is the percentage of illumination that the surface reflects. The top part of the figure indicates the reflectances of several surfaces in a visual scene. The eye responds only to changes in the intensity of the reflected light. The middle part of the figure indicates the kind of information that is generated at edges in the retinal image. Each vertical line indicates the change in intensity at an edge. The visual system integrates information from all the edges in order to reconstruct the original intensity pattern (bottom).

The visual system extracts only relative information from an edge, and such information is a small part of what the visual system needs in order to perceive color, a part that can be properly interpreted only in the context of the relative information from many other edges. There is evidence that the visual system integrates neural signals emanating from distinct edges. Recording changes in light and then integrating them is mathematically equivalent to keeping a point-by-point record of the light.

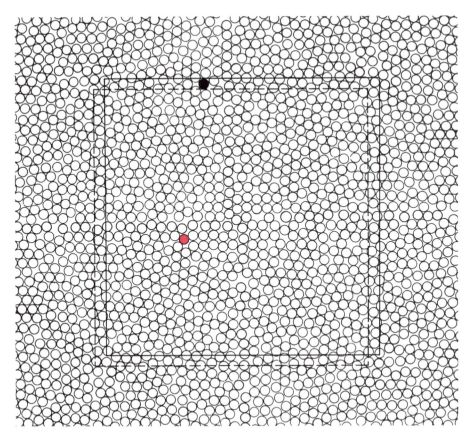

Figure 4.2 STIMULATION OF A RECEPTOR CELL (*black dot*) changes as the edge of the retinal image moves across the cell when the image shifts from one position (*solid rectangle*) to another (*broken rectangle*) because of the eye tremors. Cells, such as the colored one, that the boundary of the retinal image does not move across do not receive a change of stimulation. Since the green-red boundary in Krauskopf's display did not cross cells, the display appeared to be red.

Simply recording the changes, however, is more efficient and requires less transmission capacity. Consider an analogous situation in the stock market. To draw a graph showing how the price of a certain stock varies from day to day, one could either find out the price of the stock each day or find out the price only on days when it had changed. The latter method requires less transmission capacity, and so it might be preferred if getting the stock quotation required a transcontinental telephone call. Yet the information collected by this method could be easily integrated to give the stock prices for each day. I believe something similar to this process of information extraction and integration is going on in the visual system. Such a process has also been suggested by Edwin H. Land of the Polaroid Corpo-

ration (see Chapter 3, "The Retinex Theory of Color Vision").

It turns out, however, that the model of reflectance-edge extraction and integration is quite limited in its application. The model works well when the objects whose colors are under scrutiny are uniformly illuminated. It even works when the illumination is changing uniformly over the entire visual field, because changes in the overall illumination have no effect on the relative changes in the light at the boundary between two shades of gray. This is just a special case of the general phenomenon that a change in illumination does not change the ratio of the amount of light reflected off adjacent surfaces of differing reflectance. For example, consider two surfaces whose reflectances are respectively 25 and 50

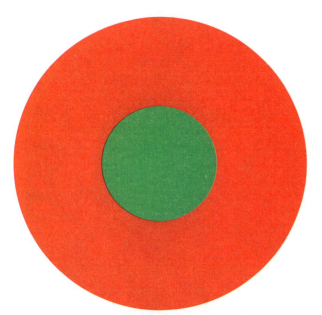 

Figure 4.3 RETINAL RECEPTOR CELLS gather color information by detecting changes in light. To detect such changes there must be constant relative displacement between the retinal image and the retina, and so the eye scans a surface by constantly flicking back and forth in tremors with a frequency of between 30 and 150 cycles per second. In the display at the left the boundary between the red ring and the green disk was moved in such a way as to follow the tremors. That eliminated all displacement between the boundary and the cells. As a result retinal boundary disappeared and observer saw a red disk (right). The experiment was done by John Krauskopf at Bell Laboratories.

percent. The ratio of reflected light will remain 1 : 2 regardless of the intensity of the illumination. It has been demonstrated that the neural signal generated at an edge in the retinal image remains the same if the intensity ratio at the edge remains the same.

The model of reflectance-edge extraction and integration runs into trouble when the objects under scrutiny are not uniformly illuminated. The trouble begins with spatial changes in the illumination. Such illumination edges are of two kinds: attached and cast (projected). Attached edges arise from changes in the planarity, or spatial orientation, of surfaces. If two walls of the same color meet at a corner and one wall receives more illumination than the other, then there is an attached illumination edge where they meet (see Figure 4.4). Such edges would also appear in a white plaster-of-Paris sculpture where irregularities in the sculpture's shape are clearly visible because the intensity of the incident illumination varies as the angle between the light source and various areas of the sculpture changes. On the other hand, the boundary of a shadow is a cast illumination edge. So is the boundary of a spotlight projected onto a stage and the boundary of a bright trapezoidal patch of light projected onto a floor by sunlight streaming through a rectangular window (see Figure 4.5).

The presence of illumination edges in the retinal image makes the simple model of reflectance-edge extraction and integration unworkable. If changes in illumination were extracted and integrated right along with reflectance changes, gross errors in perceived lightness would result. For example, a white surface in shadow might appear as a gray surface. Nevertheless, the model can be further developed to eliminate this difficulty. What is necessary is that before the edges are integrated into an intensity image they must be classified either as reflectance changes or as illumination changes. Once this classification is made, the visual system could separately integrate the two kinds of edge. The result would be two distinct images: one representing surface reflectance and the other representing surface illumination.

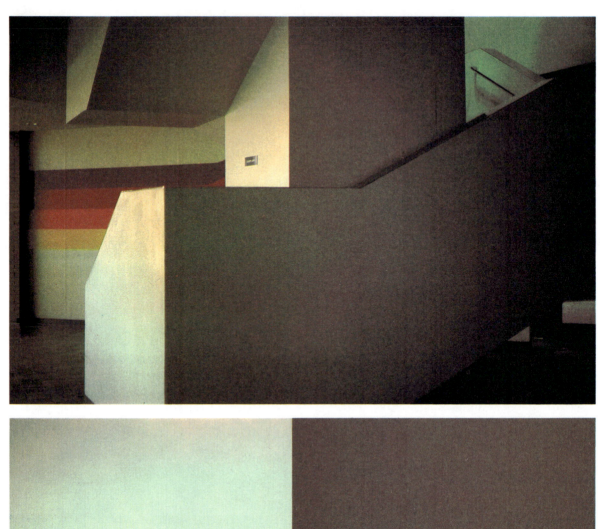

Figure 4.4 PERCEIVED SPATIAL ORIENTATION affects color perception. In the top photograph it is apparent that the right side of the stairwell is a white surface in shadow and that the left side is an illuminated white surface. Because the visual system recognizes that the stairs turn a corner it correctly perceives that the stairwell is differentially illuminated. The bottom photograph is a closeup view of the stairwell corner. Here the two sides appear to form a plane rather than a corner. The sides are perceived to be illuminated equally, and so the visual system attributes the difference in grayness to the sides themselves. Hence the shadowed side is not correctly perceived as being white.

M y own work has centered on the conditions under which the visual system can distinguish reflectance edges from illumination edges and on how the distinction might be made. I have been guided by the belief that the classification of edges cannot be carried out at the level of the retina. The fact is that spatial changes in illumination and changes in reflectance generate identical edges on the retina. Some workers have suggested that the retina could classify the edges based on their sharpness, with reflectance edges tending to be sharp and

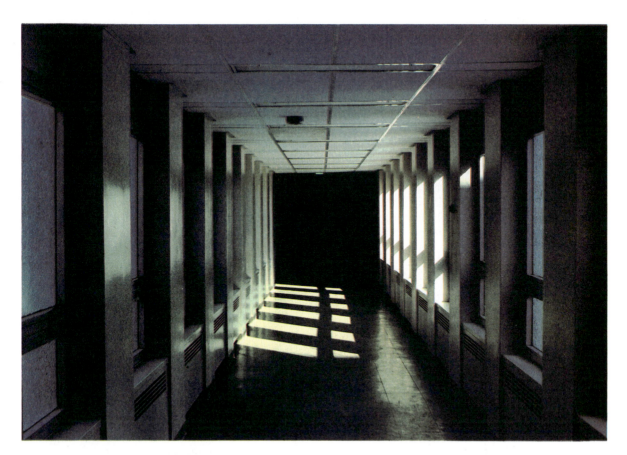

Figure 4.5 ILLUMINATION EDGES, or illumination differences, are of two kinds: attached and cast (projected). Attached edges are the result of changes in the spatial orientation of surfaces; cast edges are the result of shadows. In this photograph both kinds of edges are present in abundance. For example, there are attached edges where the walls turn corners to form the indentations that hold the windows. The boundaries of the trapezoidal patches of light projected on the floor by sunlight streaming through windows are examples of cast edges.

illumination edges tending to be gradual. This simple explanation does not work, however, because illumination edges (both cast and attached) are often sharp whereas reflectance edges are sometimes gradual. And yet the visual system can correctly identify the two kinds of edge. Rather than classifying edges solely on the basis of their sharpness on the retina the visual system must classify them on the basis of their relation to all the other edges in the entire retinal image. This means that not only the eye but also the central nervous system play a role in the classification of edges.

That the central nervous system is involved in color perception is suggested by a simple phenomenon Irvin Rock of the University of California at Berkeley pointed out to me. He noted that the shadowed side of a corner (for example, where two walls meet) usually seem to be approximately the same shade of gray as the illuminated side. When the corner is artificially made to appear flat by viewing it through a hole, however, the shadowed side seems to be an extremely dark gray, often even black. When the corner is seen this way, no shadow is perceived; the darkness is attributed to the surface itself. (Compare top and bottom photographs in Figure 4.4.)

Here is a situation where the edge at the corner can be perceived as either an illumination edge when it is seen correctly in depth or as a reflectance edge when it is made to look flat. This suggests that the visual system relies on depth information to determine whether it is the illumination or the reflectance that is changing at an edge. Moreover, the situation seems to challenge the prevailing view that lightness is determined by intensity ratios between adjacent regions of the retinal image independently of where these regions are perceived to be in three-dimensional space. To demonstrate conclusively that depth perception (and hence the central nervous system) plays a role in color perception, I tried to reproduce the corner phenomenon under strict laboratory conditions.

I suspended in midair from a hidden support two white surfaces that met to form an outside right-angled corner. Behind the surfaces I put a uniform background of medium intensity. One of the white surfaces received 30 times more light than the other surface. Observers viewed the display and indicated the apparent lightness of each surface by selecting a matching sample from a chart of various shades of gray. A second group of observers viewed the surfaces when they were made to seem flat by being looked at through a hole with one eye.

When the two surfaces looked flat, the difference in intensity was perceived as a difference in reflectance, as I had expected. In other words, the illuminated side (a value of 30) looked white and the shadowed side (a value of 1) looked black. To my surprise, however, the observers saw exactly the same thing when the surfaces appeared to be at right angles to each other. This is essentially what earlier investigators had found in similar circumstances. In a few studies the perceived spatial pattern had been found to have a small effect on perceived lightness, but in most other studies, including my own, there was no such effect.

I was so impressed by the strength of the effect of spatial orientation under natural conditions that I felt something significant about the natural context of the corner must have been lost in my attempt to reproduce the situation in the laboratory. I tried in several ways to enrich the context of the laboratory display. For example, I placed objects in the vicinity of the suspended corner so as to make the lighting conditions manifest to the observers. All these attempts failed to change the results.

Finally I found the effect of spatial orientation when I put a black surface next to and coplanar with each of the original white surfaces. As in the original display, the 30 : 1 ratio in intensity between the white surfaces was seen as a difference in reflectance when they appeared to be coplanar. When the two surfaces were seen at right angles to each other, the same intensity ratio was perceived as an illumination difference. In other words, when the surfaces were seen as being coplanar, the illuminated surface looked white and the shadowed surface looked black, but when the surfaces were seen as an outside corner, the shadowed surface was seen correctly as a white surface in shadow.

A reasonable interpretation of these results is that the visual system operates to account for the entire pattern of retinal intensities as generated by either changes in illumination or changes in reflectance. The original two-surface display could be seen as being uniformly illuminated because the two intensity levels (30 and 1) could be treated as resulting from different shades of gray, namely white (30) and black (1). The more complex four-surface display involves a 900 : 1 range of intensities. (The illuminated white surface is 900 times more intense than the shadowed black surface.) Since the range in intensity of shades of gray that can result solely from reflectance is normally limited to 30:1, the four-surface display also requires the perception of some variations in illumination. Which edges will be treated as representing illumination changes and which as representing reflectance changes depends on the overall organization of the scene, particularly the perceived three-dimensional layout.

Next I modified the four-surface display to rule out the possibility that the results were caused by some kind of contrast effect operating between adjacent areas of the two-dimensional retinal image. The horizontal plane of the modified display consisted of a large white square attached to a small black trapezoidal tab that extended outward toward

the observer (see Figure 4.6). The vertical plane consisted of a large black square attached to a small white tab that extended upward. In other words, the tabs extended out into midair from the corner formed by the two large squares, and so each tab appears on three sides against a background that is not in the same plane. As in the original four-surface display, the horizontal plane received 30 times more light than the vertical plane. The tabs are trapezoidal in order to create an illusion in depth perception.

Seen with both eyes the tabs correctly appear as trapezoids lying in their actual planes. In this case the vertical tab appears to be almost white and the horizontal tab almost black. On the other hand, seen through an aperture with only one eye each trapezoidal tab appears to be a small square lying in

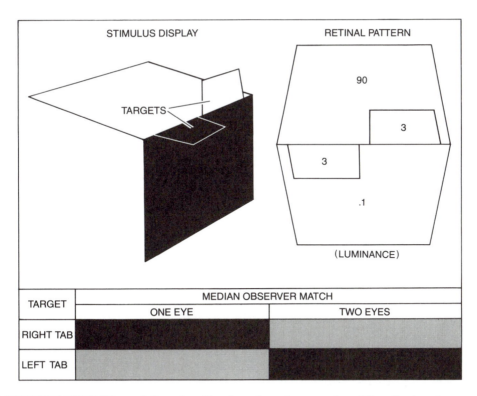

Figure 4.6 STIMULUS DISPLAY, consisting of an illuminated horizontal plane and a shadowed vertical plane, was viewed by observers who looked down at it from an angle of 45 degrees. Because the targets were trapezoids each seemed to lie in the same plane as one of the larger background squares when the display was viewed with one eye through an aperture. When the targets were viewed with both eyes, they were seen in their actual spatial positions. In both cases the retinal pattern remained the same, although the perceived lightness changed. The chart indicates what the observers saw.

the same plane as the larger square that surrounds it on three sides. In this case the perceived colors are the reverse: the vertical tab appears to be black and the horizontal tab appears to be white.

In both cases, however, the retinal image is the same: each tab is seen against a square background that surrounds it on three sides. This means that the relation between the target and its background in the retinal image is irrelevant to the target's perceived shade of gray. The shade of gray turns out to depend on the relation between the intensity of the target and the intensity of whatever surface seems to lie in the same plane, even if that coplanar surface does not provide the background of the target in the retinal image. Therefore when the display is seen with both eyes, the shadowed white vertical tab appears to be coplanar with the shadowed black vertical background, and so the tab appears to be white. In addition the illuminated black horizontal tab appears to be coplanar with the illuminated white horizontal background, and so the tab looks black. When the display is seen with one eye, the shadowed white vertical tab appears to be coplanar with the illuminated white horizontal background, and so the tab looks black. Moreover, the illuminated black horizontal tab appears to be coplanar with the shadowed black vertical background, and so the tab looks white.

The model of edge extraction, classification and integration was put to a more direct test in a series of experiments designed to probe what observers would see if a reflectance edge were mistakenly perceived as an illumination edge or vice versa. The corner experiments I have described showed that a change in the perceived type of edge results in a change in the perceived lightness of the region bounded by the perceptually altered edge. If perceived lightness depends on the visual system's integration of a series of spatially remote edges, then even stranger perceptual mistakes will manifest themselves. For example, if a single reflectance edge in a complex display is made to appear as an illumination edge, then in certain circumstances this ought to have as great an effect on the perceived lightness of regions that are remote from the altered edge as it has on the regions that are bounded by the altered edge.

At the State University of New York at Stony Brook, Stanley Delman and I designed one such edge-substitution experiment. We studied a familiar

display, known as simultaneous lightness contrast, that is often treated in psychology textbooks. Two middle-gray squares are placed respectively on adjacent white and black backgrounds (see Figure 4.7a). It turns out that for some reason the gray square on the white background looks slightly darker than the gray square on the black background. This effect, however, was not the subject of our experiment. We wanted to reproduce the same pattern of reflected light that the eye receives from this display when the boundary between the white and black backgrounds was perceived as the boundary between high and low levels of illumination.

To this end we affixed to a wall a large rectangular piece of middle-gray paper that would serve as the immediate background for both target squares. The difference in immediate background intensities was created by casting a beam of light with a sharp edge across half of the gray rectangle. Part of the beam also illuminated the background wall on three sides of the rectangle. The intensity of the beam was set so that the intensity ratio of the illuminated half of the gray rectangle to the shadowed half was 30:1, which is equal to the intensity ratio of white paper to black paper, as was the case in the original display. Next we needed to add the target squares. They could not be the same shade of gray (that is, have the same reflectance), because they would then reflect different amounts of light to the eye owing to their unequal illumination.

In the original lightness-contrast display that we were trying to reproduce the two squares reflected exactly the same amount of light. It is also true that in the original display the squares had the same reflectance. That did not concern us, however, because our goal was to reproduce not all the facets of the original display but only the information the visual system received: the pattern of light intensities that reached the eye. To achieve this goal the target square on the shadowed side had to have a reflectance 30 times as great as the other target square, which would be receiving 30 times as much illumination. Therefore we placed a white square on the shadowed side and a black square on the illuminated side (see Figure 4.7c).

In this way we thought we had reproduced in a logical manner the light intensities of the original pattern (see Figure 4.7b). Now it was time to test our results photometrically and empirically. Photometric measurements showed that the targets reflected

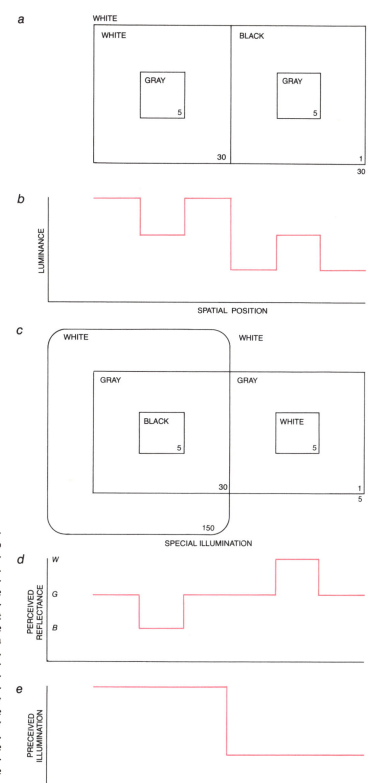

Figure 4.7 LIGHTNESS-CONTRAST DISPLAY (*a*) gives rise to an intensity pattern (*b*) that consists solely of reflectance edges. The two gray squares are perceived as being almost the same shade of middle gray. The identical intensity pattern can result from an illumination difference and an altered display (*c*). When observers viewed the display, they could clearly see that a rectangular beam of light was illuminating half of it (*e*), and so the illuminated target was correctly perceived as being black and the shadowed target was correctly perceived as being white (*d*). When seen through an aperture that revealed only the gray rectangle, the display looked like the original reflectance display.

equal amounts of light, that the immediate background on one side reflected 30 times more light than the immediate background on the other side and that on a logarithmic scale the target intensities were halfway between the intensities of the two immediate backgrounds. All of this was true of the original display as well. Moreover, the reproduction preserved the geometry of the original.

Empirical considerations also indicated that our reproduction was faithful. Under control conditions observers viewed our reproduction through a rectangular aperture in a cardboard screen. The screen limited the observers' view so that the only parts of the display that were visible were the two square targets and their immediate backgrounds: the illuminated and shadowed halves of the gray rectangle. Under these conditions the display looked just like the original. The immediate backgrounds looked respectively white and black even though they were actually a middle gray that had been differentially illuminated. The illumination edge between the immediate backgrounds was perceived as a reflectance edge, and the square targets looked middle gray, one slightly darker than the other.

All of this served merely to assure us that we had correctly reproduced the pattern of light reflected by the original display. The real test came when we had observers view the display without looking through the confining cardboard screen. Under these conditions the observers could clearly see that a beam of light was illuminating half of the rectangular piece of paper since the beam of light illuminated the part of the background wall that was behind this half of the rectangle. Now the illuminated target was correctly perceived as black whereas the shadowed target was correctly perceived as white (see Figure 4.7d and e).

The perceived lightness of each target changed radically from the screened display to the unscreened one in spite of the fact that the amount of light each target reflected remained the same, that the amount of light each immediate background reflected remained the same and hence that the neural signal generated at the retinal edge of each immediate background must have remained the same. This clearly means that color perception is not simply a function of the amount of light a surface reflects, of the intensity ratio of a surface to its immediate background or of the neural signal generated at the retinal edge of a surface.

It seems that a much more relativistic process is going on in the visual system. The boundary between each target square and its immediate background gives only the relation between the light reflected by each of these areas. If one target is to be compared with the other, the relation between the immediate backgrounds must be taken into account. If the immediate backgrounds are perceived to differ radically in reflectance, then this perception, together with the edges between the targets and the backgrounds, suggests that the targets are nearly the same in lightness. If, on the other hand, the immediate backgrounds are perceived to differ radically in illumination, then the targets appear to lie against the same (reflectance) background and hence appear to differ extremely in lightness.

It is now time to consider how the model of edge classification incorporates the above results. In the screened case where the display looked like the original lightness-contrast display the changes at the edges could simply be extracted and integrated to form an intensity profile of the display. In the unscreened case the same intensity profile would be generated if the edges were not classified either as illumination edges or as reflectance edges. If, however, the edges are classified before the integration, and if the integration is done only within each class of edges, then two separate profiles are generated. In that case the reflectance profile of the screened display should be different from the reflectance profile of the unscreened one. The difference is that the middle edge representing the relation between the immediate backgrounds is present only in the reflectance profile of the screened display. This means that in the unscreened display the targets look sharply different in reflectance (namely as white and as black) rather than appearing to be two shades of middle gray. Of course, the edge between the immediate backgrounds that is missing from the reflectance profile would manifest itself in the illumination profile. Thus the illumination profile would show a region of high illumination next to a region of low illumination. In the screened display the illumination profile would simply be uniform.

Alfred Yarbus of the Academy of Sciences of the U.S.S.R. did a similar experiment using the technique by which the image on the retina is stabilized even as the eye moves back and forth [and showed that a change in information at an edge affects regions that are spatially remote from the altered edge]. He placed a white and a black region next to each other on a red background (see Figure 4.8). Disk-shaped targets of the same shade of red as the background were placed in the center of both the white and the black region. Under normal viewing conditions the disk on the white region would look slightly darker than the disk on the black region. Yarbus altered the conditions so as to eliminate the perceptual boundaries between the white and the black region and between these regions and the red background. This he accomplished with an apparatus that caused the physical boundaries to move along with the eye, as Krauskopf had done with his green disk and red annulus. Since the eye registers only changes in light intensity when there is constant relative displacement between the retinal image and the retina, it could not detect the presence of the white and black regions. As a result the disks appeared to stand on a homogeneous red background. Yarbus did not report his results quantitatively, but he indicated that one disk (the one objectively on the white region) appeared very dark whereas the other disk appeared very light.

Yarbus' results were essentially the same as mine, although there were significant differences in our respective methods. In Yarbus' experiment and in my unscreened display the targets were made to look as though they had a common background by removing from the reflectance profile the edge that partitioned the background. As far as perceived lightness goes the effects are the same. What is fascinating is that Yarbus removed the edge at the point of extraction, whereas I removed the edge at the point of classification. To put it another way, in Yarbus' experiment the eye never detects the edge, whereas in my unscreened display the eye detects it and then classifies it correctly as an illumination edge. In Yarbus' experiment there is no reason to believe the observers saw the targets as being differentially illuminated.

Yarbus' experiment gives direct evidence for the validity of the concept of edge extraction and integration. The edge of each disk did not change; rather, boundaries that partitioned the background disappeared. As with Krauskopf's green disk and red annulus, the region bounded by the disappearing edge seemed to change color. Here the white and black regions of the background disappeared, leaving only a single uniformly colored background. Yarbus' work, however, reveals an additional phenomenon: the disks appeared to change color even though their boundaries remained constantly visible. The obvious conclusion is that information at one edge (here the edge between a disk and its

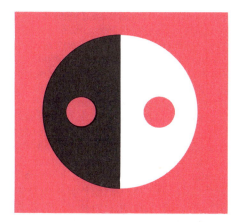 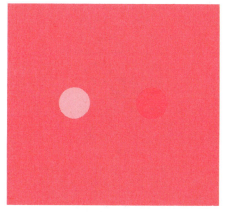

Figure 4.8 OBSERVERS viewed the display at the left under conditions where the white and black backgrounds were not perceived because the boundary between them and the boundaries between each of them and the surrounding red background were moved back and forth to follow eye tremors. The target disks appeared to lie on a homogeneously red background (*right*) where the bound- **ary of the disk at the right still carried the information that the disk was darker than its immediate background and therefore appeared dark red. The boundary of the disk at the left still carried the information that the disk was lighter than its immediate background, so that it appeared a very light red.**

immediate background and the surrounding background) is integrated in some way with the information at a remote edge (here the edge between the immediate background and the surrounding background) before the color of any region is finally perceived.

It would be helpful at this point to discuss why the visual system determines surface colors by comparing intensities of reflected light. As I have mentioned, making such a comparison involves extracting information from edges. This suggests that it is more useful to think of the retinal image as a pattern of edges than it is to think of it as a mosaic of color patches, as traditional accounts of color perception would have it. The edges are of two kinds, and so the retinal image is actually a dual image.

The retina is a light-sensitive surface designed to register gradients in the optic array. There are basically two kinds of change in the physical world that result in gradients of stimulation on the retina: change in surface reflectance and change in illumination. Each kind of change is capable by itself of producing a complex pattern of stimulation on the retina. From a large expanse of uniformly illuminated wallpaper the retina receives a pattern arising solely from changes in surface reflectance. On the other hand, from the rumpled white sheets of an unmade bed or from a snow-covered landscape the retina receives a pattern of stimulation arising solely out of changes in illumination. Normally these two kinds of change are at work simultaneously. It is as if two separate patterns have been laid on top of each other on the retina. The task of the visual system is to disentangle the two patterns.

The duality of the retinal image implies that each point in the visual system has at least two values: a reflectance value and an illumination value. The perception of transparency involves a similar two-value phenomenon, because a surface of one color is seen behind a surface of another color. The same phenomenon is involved in reflections. For example, when an observer looks through a window, the observer sees two scenes at once: the actual scene outside the window and another scene reflected on the inside of the window. As a result it is possible to see two colors in the same place.

Consider an experience I had recently. A book with a red cover had been left on top of the dashboard of my car in such a way that I could see a red reflection of the book as I looked out through the windshield. I was surprised to find that distant objects retained their normal colors as they were viewed through the red reflection. Even green objects seen through the red reflection looked green. This interested me because I of course knew that when red and green light are mixed in isolation, they form yellow. Then when I held up my hand to block the rest of the scene and viewed just a patch of the red and green through a small opening between my fingers, I did see yellow. The opening in my hand had imposed the same boundary on the red and green light, and so they mixed to form yellow. In the original situation, however, the boundary of the red reflection did not coincide with the boundary of the green object. As a result the red and the green light appeared as elements of separate images rather than as yellow. Apparently when one speaks of mixing colors, one should actually speak of mixing edges (changes in the light) rather than of mixing light itself.

Such considerations indicate that the retina does not act as a photocell in measuring the intensity and color at each point in a scene. Man-made measuring devices are designed to respond to only one physical quantity at a time. For example, if a voltmeter is sensitive to resistance or, worse, to temperature, the meter is considered defective. To cite such devices as models of the human sensory system can be extremely misleading. Unlike man-made measuring devices, the human visual system seems capable of processing multiple variables simultaneously. Accounts of color perception relying on inappropriate measuring-device models maintain that the visual system gains information about surface reflectance by sacrificing information about illumination. Such accounts unnecessarily limit the visual system to simple situations, when in fact it can handle complex situations by extracting information about changes in reflectance and illumination.

I have discussed how the visual system deals with retinal images composed of both reflectance edges and illumination edges. It is also possible to study the perception of images that show only one kind of edge. I wondered how things would look if all the reflectance edges were missing from a situation. Alan Jacobsen and I built two miniature rooms that consisted entirely of illumination edges. We furnished each room identically with the same number of objects of varying size and shape. We painted one room, including all its contents, a matte (non-glossy) white, and we painted the other matte black. Observers viewed each room through an aperture in one of its walls, which prevented them from seeing the light bulb that illuminated the room.

It is important to keep in mind that each of these rooms projects a complex nonuniform pattern of stimulation on the retina of the observer. In the room there are sharp edges at corners and fuzzier ones across walls and curved surfaces. Some of the edges are the result of cast shadows, but all of them are illumination edges, since we eliminated the reflectance edges by covering everything with paint of a single reflectance.

In presenting these displays to naïve observers we had a number of questions in mind. We wondered whether the edges in the room would be perceived as changes in reflectance, as prevailing theories of lightness perception would predict, or as changes in illumination, as the changes actually were. In other words, would each room be correctly perceived as a single shade of gray? And if it was so perceived, what shade of gray would it be? Would the black room look black and the white room white?

It turns out that 22 of our 24 observers saw each room as being uniform in lightness. They had correctly attributed the variations in intensity to variations in illumination. All of them saw the white room as white. As for the black room, all of them saw it as consisting of only a single shade of gray, although the perceived shade varied from observer to observer. The shades ranged from black to middle gray and averaged to a dark gray.

The model of edge extraction, classification and integration suggested that the illumination edges in the two rooms would be perceived as such and hence that the reflectance of each room would seem uniform. Yet there is nothing in the model so far to predict that observers could identify at least roughly the correct shade of gray. What information makes this identification possible? A plausible hypothesis is that the identification is made on the basis of the intensity of the light. In our experiment the average intensity of the light reflected from the white room is higher than the average intensity of the light reflected from the black room. By modifying our experiment, however, we invalidated the hypothesis. We lowered the intensity of the light source in the white room and raised the intensity of that in the black room until every point in the black room

reflected more light than the corresponding point in the white room. The results were the same: the white room looked white and the black room looked dark gray.

We now have a promising lead to how the visual system determines the shade of gray in these rooms, although we do not yet have a complete explanation. (John Robinson helped me to develop this lead.) We believe the operative factor is the effect of indirect illumination on the retinal pattern. Every point in our rooms received illumination from two sources: directly from the light bulb and indirectly from light reflected from other surfaces in the room. In the black room, which had a reflectance of about 3 percent, there was scarcely any indirect illumination. Direct light accounted for almost all the light shining on the various surfaces. Direct light generates sharp edges, and so the intensity profile of the black room revealed a wild pattern of up-and-down swings. Although the relative pattern of direct illumination turned out to be the same in the two rooms, there was much more indirect illumination in the white room, whose reflectance was about 90 percent. Such abundant indirect light had the effect of smearing out the sharp edges resulting from the direct illumination, so that the intensity profile of the white room revealed a smoother pattern of gradual changes (see Figure 4.9).

When we reduced the illumination in the white room, the shape of the intensity profile did not change. The profile merely showed a uniform decrease in intensity. If the white room were painted a darker shade of gray, the shape of its profile would change. Our work demonstrates that black rooms have sharper gradients than white rooms. In some way the visual system deciphers the shade of gray of a room from the shape of the intensity pattern of the room. Our work in this area is only at the beginning. As we learn more about the information stored in the intensity pattern, we hope to understand the deciphering process.

My co-workers and I have begun to extend our analysis of shades of gray to the chromatic colors. In one experiment we compared the observations of subjects who viewed a white room illuminated with blue light with the observations of those who viewed a blue room illuminated with white light. All the subjects were able to tell whether the blue-

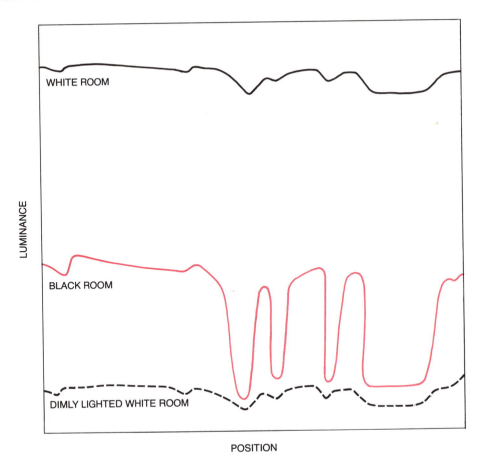

Figure 4.9 INDIRECT ILLUMINATIONS may affect how the visual system determines grayness. Curves depict the intensity profiles of the same furnished room painted entirely white (*top*), painted white but dimly lighted (*bottom*) and painted black (*middle*). In the white room, the intensity profiles (*top and bottom*) are comparatively smooth. In the black room, there was very little indirect illumination, so that the profile (*middle*) revealed a pattern of up-and-down swings characteristic of edges generated by direct illumination. Perceived grayness does not depend on the intensity of reflected light, since the black room reflected more light than the dimly lighted white room.

ness came from the surfaces or from the illumination, in spite of the fact that the light reflected off corresponding patches in the two rooms might be identical. This result clearly indicates that the perception of illumination also plays an important role in the perception of chromatic surface color.

The question of whether or not surface-color perception can be explained without reference to the perception of illumination has been debated since the end of the 19th century, when Hermann von Helmholtz first proposed that surface color could be determined only after illumination had been estimated. Helmholtz, however, was unable to specify how the illumination is estimated, so that most accounts of color perception have failed to refer to perceived illumination. The experiments I have described here suggest that Helmholtz was correct in his emphasis on perceived illumination but incorrect in his ideas about its relation to perceived surface color. He assumed incorrectly that the eye measures light. Current work shows that the eye compares light by extracting edge information, and so the visual system acquires information about illumination in exactly the same way that it acquires information about the colors of the surfaces in a scene. It turns out that the perception of illumination and the perception of surface color are parallel processes in the visual system involving the decomposition of the retinal image into separate patterns of illumination and surface color.

INFORMATION PROCESSING

. . .

Vision by Man and Machine

How does an animal see? How might a computer do it? A study of stereo vision guides research on both these questions. Brain science suggests computer programs; the computer suggests what to look for in the brain.

. . .

Tomaso Poggio
April, 1984

The development of computers of increasing power and sophistication often stimulates comparisons between them and the human brain, and these comparisons are becoming more earnest as computers are applied more and more to tasks formerly associated with essentially human activities and capabilities. Indeed, it is widely expected that a coming generation of computers and robots will have sensory, motor and even "intellectual" skills closely resembling our own. How might such machines be designed? Can our rapidly growing knowledge of the human brain be a guide? And at the same time can our advances in "artificial intelligence" help us to understand the brain?

At the level of their hardware (the brain's or a computer's) the differences are great. The neurons, or nerve cells, in a brain are small, delicate structures bound by a complex membrane and closely packed in a medium of supporting cells that control a complex and probably quite variable chemical environment. They are very unlike the wires and etched crystals of semiconducting materials on which computers are based. In the organization of the hardware the differences also are great. The connections between neurons are very numerous (any one neuron may receive many thousands of inputs) and are distributed in three dimensions. In a computer the wires linking circuit components are limited by present-day solid-state technology to a relatively small number arranged more or less two-dimensionally.

In the transmission of signals the differences again are great. The binary (on-off) electric pulses of the computer are mirrored to some extent in the all-or-nothing signal conducted along nerve fibers, but in addition the brain employs graded electrical signals, chemical messenger substances and the transport of ions. In temporal organization the differences are immense. Computers process information serially (one step at a time) but at a very fast rate. The time course of their operation is governed by a computer-wide clock. What is known of the brain suggests that it functions much slower but that it analyzes information along millions of channels concurrently without need of clock-driven operation.

How, then, are brains and computers alike? Clearly there must be a level at which any two mechanisms can be compared. One can compare the tasks they do. "To bring the good news from Ghent to Aix" is a description of a task that can be done by satellite, telegraph, horseback messenger or pigeon post equally well (unless other constraints such as time are specified). If, therefore, we assert that brains and computers function as information-processing systems, we can develop descriptions of the tasks they perform that will be equally applicable to either. We shall have a common language in which to discuss them: the language of information processing. Note that in this language descriptions of tasks are decoupled from descriptions of the hardware that perform them. This separability is at the foundation of the science of artificial intelligence. Its goals are to make computers more useful by endowing them with "intelligent" capabilities, and beyond that to understand the principles that make intelligence possible.

In no field have the descriptions of information-processing tasks been more precisely formulated than in the study of vision. On the one hand it is the dominant sensory modality of human beings. If we want to create robots capable of performing complex manipulative tasks in a changing environment, we must surely endow them with adequate visual powers. Yet vision remains elusive. It is something we are good at; the brain does it rapidly and easily. It is nonetheless a mammoth information-processing task. If it required a conscious effort, like adding numbers in our head, we would not undervalue its difficulty. Instead we are easily lured into oversimple, noncomputational preconceptions of what vision really entails.

Ultimately, of course, one wants to know how vision is performed by the biological hardware of neurons and their synaptic interconnections. But vision is not exclusively a problem in anatomy and physiology: how nerve cells are interconnected and how they act. From the perspective of information processing (by the brain or by a computer) it is a problem at many levels: the level of computation (What computational tasks must a visual system perform?), the level of algorithm (What sequence of steps completes the task?) and then the level of hardware (How might neurons or electronic circuits execute the algorithm?). Thus an attack on the problem of vision requires a variety of aids, including psychophysical evidence (that is, knowledge of how well people can see) and neurophysiological data (knowledge of what neurons can do). Finding workable algorithms is the most critical part of the project, because algorithms are constrained both by the computation and by the available hardware.

Figure 5.1 STEREO VISION BY A COMPUTER is shown in aerial photographs (provided by Robert J. Woodham). They were made from different angles so that objects in each have slightly different positions. The images were made by a mosaic of microelectronic sensors, each of which measures the intensity of light along a particular line of sight, as do the photoreceptor cells of the eye. The map at the bottom was generated by a computer programmed to follow a procedure devised by David Marr and the author and further developed by W. Eric L. Grimson. The computer filtered the images to emphasize spatial changes in intensity. Then it performed stereopsis: it matched features from one image to the other, determined the disparity between their positions and calculated their relative depths in the three-dimensional world. Increasing elevations in the map are coded in colors from blue to red.

Here I shall outline an effort in which I am involved, one that explores a sequence of algorithms first to extract information, notably edges, or pronounced contours in the intensity of light, from visual images and then to calculate from those edges the depths of objects in the three-dimensional world. I shall concentrate on a particular aspect of the task, namely stereopsis, or stereo vision (see Figure 5.1). Not the least of my reasons is the central role stereopsis has played in the work on vision that my colleagues and I have done at the Artificial Intelligence Laboratory of the Massachusetts Institute of Technology. In particular, stereopsis has stimulated a close investigation of the very first steps in visual information processing. Then too, stereopsis is deceptively simple. As with so many other tasks that the brain performs without effort, the development of an automatic system with stereo vision has proved to be surprisingly difficult. Finally, the study of stereopsis benefits from the availability of a large body of psychophysical evidence that defines and constrains the problem.

The information available at the outset of the process of vision is a two-dimensional array of measurements of the amount of light reflected into the eye or into a camera from points on the surfaces of objects in the three-dimensional visual world. In the human eye the measurements are made by photoreceptors (rod cells and cone cells), of which there are more than 100 million. In a camera that my colleagues and I use at the Artificial Intelligence Laboratory the processes are different but the result is much the same. There the measurements are made by solid-state electronic sensors. They pro-

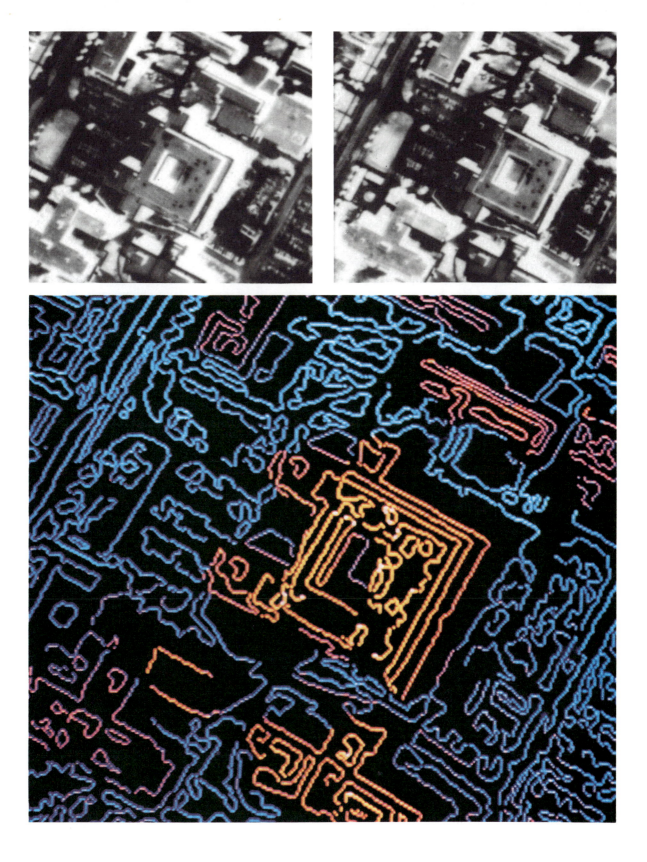

duce an array of 1,000 by 1,000 light-intensity values. Each value is a pixel, or picture element (see Figure 5.2).

In either case it is inconceivable that the gap between the raw image (the large array of numbers produced by the eye or the camera) and vision (knowing *what* is around, and *where*) can be spanned in a single step. One concludes that vision requires various processes—one thinks of them as modules—operating in parallel on raw images and producing intermediate representations of the images on which other processes can work. For example, several vision modules seem to be involved in reconstructing the three-dimensional geometry of the world. A short list of such modules would have to include modules that deduce shape from shading, from visual texture, from motion, from contours, from occlusions and from stereopsis. Some may work directly on the raw image (the intensity measurements). Often, however, a module may operate more effectively on an intermediate representation.

Stereopsis arises from the fact that our two eyes view the visual world from slightly different angles. To put it another way, the eyes converge slightly, so that their axes of vision meet at a point in the visual world. The point is said to be fixated by the eyes, that is, the image of the point falls on the center of vision of each retina. Any neighboring point in the visual field will then project to a point on each retina some distance from the center of vision. In general this distance will not be the same for both eyes. In fact, the disparity in distance will vary with the depth of the point in the visual field with respect to the fixated point (see Figure 5.3).

Stereopsis, then, is the decoding of three-dimensionality from binocular disparities. It might appear at first to be a straightforward problem in trigonometry. One might therefore be tempted to program a computer to solve it that way. The effort would fail; our own facility with stereopsis has led us to gloss over the central difficulty of the task, as we may see if we formally set out the steps involved in the task. They are four: A location in space must be selected from one retinal image. The same location must be identified in the other retinal image. Their positions must be measured. From the disparity between the two measurements the distance to the location must be calculated.

The last two steps are indeed an exercise in trigonometry (at least in the cases considered in this chapter). The first two steps are different. They require, in effect, that the projection of the same point in the physical world be found in each eye. A group of contiguous photoreceptors in one eye can be thought of as looking along a line of sight to a patch of the surface of some object. The photoreceptors looking at the same patch of surface from the opposite eye must then be identified. Because of binocular disparity they will not be at the same position with respect to the center of vision.

This, of course, is where the difficulty lies. For us the visual world contains surfaces that seem effectively labeled because they belong to distinct shapes in specific spatial relations to one another. One must remember, however, that vision begins with no more than arrays of raw light intensity measured from point to point. Could it be that the brain matches patterns of raw light intensity from one eye to the other? Probably not. Experiments with computers place limits on the effectiveness of the matching, and physiological and psychophysical evidence speaks against it for the human visual system. For one thing, a given patch of surface will not necessarily reflect the same intensity of light to both eyes. More important, patches of surface widely separated in the visual world may happen to have the same intensity. Matching such patches would be incorrect.

A discovery made at AT&T Bell Laboratories by Bela Julesz (now at Rutgers University) shows the full extent of the problem. Julesz devised pairs of what he called random-dot stereograms. They are visual stimuli that contain no perceptual clues except binocular disparities. To make each pair he generated a random texture of black and white dots and made two copies of it. In one of the copies he shifted an area of the pattern, say a square. In the other copy he shifted the square in the opposite direction. He filled the resulting hole in each pattern with more random texture. Viewed one at a time each pattern looked uniformly random (see Figure 5.4). Viewed through a stereoscope, so that each eye saw one of the patterns and the brain could fuse the two, the result was startling. The square gave a vivid impression of floating in front of its surroundings or behind them (see Figure 5.5). Evidently stereopsis does not require the prior perception of objects or the recognition of shapes.

Julesz' discovery enables one to formulate the computational goal of stereopsis: it is the extraction of binocular disparities from a pair of images

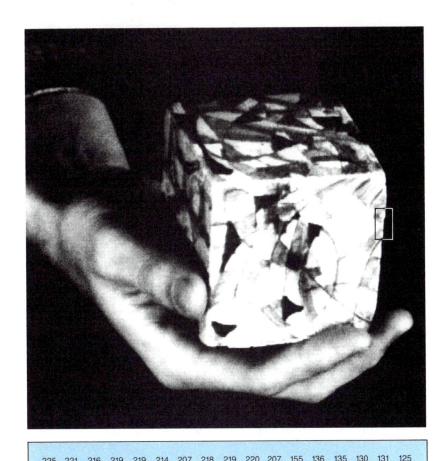

225	221	216	219	219	214	207	218	219	220	207	155	136	135	130	131	125
213	206	213	223	208	217	223	221	223	216	195	156	141	130	128	138	123
206	217	210	216	224	223	228	230	234	216	207	157	136	132	137	130	128
211	213	221	223	220	222	237	216	219	220	176	149	137	132	125	136	121
216	210	231	227	224	228	231	210	195	227	181	141	131	133	131	124	122
223	229	218	230	228	214	213	209	198	224	161	140	133	127	133	122	133
220	219	224	220	219	215	215	206	206	221	159	143	133	131	129	127	127
221	215	211	214	220	218	221	212	218	204	148	141	131	130	128	129	118
214	211	211	218	214	220	226	216	223	209	143	141	141	124	121	132	125
211	208	223	213	216	226	231	230	241	199	153	141	136	125	131	125	136
200	224	219	215	217	224	232	241	240	211	150	139	128	132	129	124	132
204	206	208	205	233	241	241	252	242	192	151	141	133	130	127	129	129
200	205	201	216	232	248	255	246	231	210	149	141	132	126	134	128	139
191	194	209	238	245	255	249	235	238	197	146	139	130	132	129	132	123
189	199	200	227	239	237	235	236	247	192	145	142	124	133	125	138	128
198	196	209	211	210	215	236	240	232	177	142	137	135	124	129	132	128
198	203	205	208	211	224	226	240	210	160	139	132	129	130	122	124	131
216	209	214	220	210	231	245	219	169	143	148	129	128	136	124	128	123
211	210	217	218	214	227	244	221	162	140	139	129	133	131	122	126	128
215	210	216	216	209	220	248	200	156	139	131	129	139	128	123	130	128
219	220	211	208	205	209	240	217	154	141	127	130	124	142	134	128	129
229	224	212	214	220	229	234	208	151	145	128	128	142	122	126	132	124
252	224	222	224	233	244	228	213	143	141	135	128	131	129	128	124	131
255	235	230	249	253	240	228	193	147	139	132	128	136	125	125	128	119
250	245	238	245	246	235	235	190	139	136	134	135	126	130	126	137	132
240	238	233	232	235	255	246	168	156	141	129	127	136	134	135	130	126
241	242	225	219	225	255	255	183	139	141	126	139	128	137	128	128	130
234	218	221	217	211	252	242	166	144	139	132	130	128	129	127	121	132
231	221	219	214	218	225	238	171	145	141	124	134	131	134	131	126	131
228	212	214	214	213	208	209	159	134	136	139	134	126	127	127	124	122
219	213	215	215	205	215	222	161	135	141	128	129	131	128	125	128	127

Figure 5.2 BEGINNING OF VISION for an animal or a computer is a gray-level array: a point-by-point representation of the intensity of light produced by a grid of detectors in the eye or in a digital camera. The image at the top of this illustration is such an array. It was produced by a digital camera as a set of intensity values in a grid of 576 by 454 picture elements ("pixels"). Intensity values for the part of the image inside the rectangle are given digitally at the bottom. (Figures 5.2 and 5.6 were prepared by H. Keith Nishihara of the Artificial Intelligence Laboratory.)

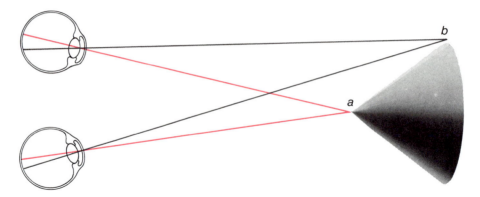

Figure 5.3 BINOCULAR DISPARITIES are the basis for stereopsis. They arise because the eyes converge slightly, so that their axes of vision meet at a point in the external world (*a*). The point is "fixated." A neighboring point in the world (*b*) will then project to a point on the retina some distance from the center of vision. The distance will not be the same for each eye.

without the need for obvious monocular clues. In addition the discovery enables one to formulate the computational problem inherent in stereopsis. It is the correspondence problem: the matching of elements in the two images that correspond to the same location in space without the recognition of objects or their parts. In random-dot stereograms the black dots in each image are all the same: they have the same size, the same shape and the same brightness. Any one of them could in principle be matched with any one of a great number of dots in the other image. And yet the brain solves this false-target dilemma: it consistently chooses only the correct set of matches.

It must use more than the dots themselves. In particular, the fact that the brain can solve the correspondence problem shows it exploits a set of implicit assumptions about the visual world, assumptions that constrain the correspondence problem, making it determined and solvable. In 1976 David Marr and I, working at MIT, found that simple properties of physical surfaces could limit the problem sufficiently for the stereopsis algorithms (procedures to be followed by a computer) we were then investigating. These are, first, that a given point on a physical surface has only one three-dimensional location at any given time and, second, that physical objects are cohesive and usually are opaque, so that the variation in depth over a surface is generally smooth, with discontinuous changes occurring only at boundary lines. The first of these constraints— uniqueness of location—means that each item in

either image (say each dot in a random-dot stereogram) has a unique disparity and can be matched with no more than one item in the other image. The second constraint—continuity and opacity— means that disparity varies smoothly except at object boundaries.

Together the two constraints provide matching rules that are reasonable and powerful. I shall describe some simple ones below. Before that, however, it is necessary to specify the items to be matched. After all, the visual world is not a random-dot stereogram, consisting only of black and white dots. We have already seen that intensity values are too unreliable. Yet the information the brain requires is encrypted in the intensity array provided by photoreceptors. If an additional property of physical surfaces is invoked, the problem is simplified. It is based on the observation that at places where there are physical changes in a surface, the image of the surface usually shows sharp variations in intensity. These variations (caused by markings on a surface and by variations in its depth) would be more reliable tokens for matching than raw intensities would be.

Instead of raw numerical values of intensity, therefore, one seeks a more symbolic, compact and robust representation of the visual world: a description of the world in which the primitive symbols— the signs in which the visual world is coded—are intensity variations. Marr called it a "primal sketch." In essence it is the conversion of the gray-level arrays provided by the visual photoreceptors

Figure 5.4 RANDOM-DOT STEREOGRAMS devised by Bela Julesz working at AT&T Bell Laboratories are visual textures containing no clues for stereo vision except binocular disparities. The stereograms themselves are the same random texture of black and white dots (*top*). In one of them, however, a square of the texture is shifted toward the left; in the other it is shifted toward the right (*bottom*). The resulting hole in each image is filled with more random dots (*gray areas*).

into a form that makes explicit the position, direction, scale and magnitude of significant light-intensity gradients, with which the brain's stereopsis module can solve the correspondence problem and reconstruct the three-dimensional geometry of the visual world. I shall describe a scheme we have been using at the Artificial Intelligence Laboratory for the past few years, based on old and new ideas developed by a number of investigators, primarily Marr, Ellen C. Hildreth and me. It has several attractive features: it is fairly simple, it works well and it shows interesting resemblances to biological vision, which, in fact, suggested it. It is not, however, the full solution. Perhaps it is best seen as a working hypothesis about vision.

Basically the changes of intensity in an image can be detected by comparing neighboring intensity values in the image: if the difference between them is great, the intensity is changing rapidly. In mathematical terms the operation amounts to taking the first derivative. (The first derivative is simply the rate of change of a mathematical function. Here it is simply the rate at which intensity changes on a path across the gray-level array.) The position of an extremal value—a peak or a pit—in the first deriva-

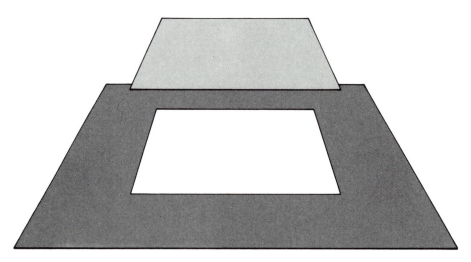

Figure 5.5 VIVID PERCEPTION OF DEPTH results when the random-dot stereograms shown in Figure 5.4 are viewed through a stereoscope, so that each eye sees one of the pair and the brain can fuse the two. The sight of part of the image "floating" establishes that stereopsis does not require the recognition of objects in the visual world.

tive turns out to localize the position of an intensity edge quite well (see Figure 5.6) In turn the intensity edge often corresponds to an edge on a physical surface. The second derivative also serves well. It is simply the rate of change of the rate of change and is obtained by taking differences between neighboring values of the first derivative. In the second derivative an intensity edge in the gray-level array corresponds to a zero-crossing: a place where the second derivative crosses zero as it falls from positive values to negative values or rises from negative values to positive.

Derivatives seem quite promising. Used alone, however, they seldom work on a real image, largely because the intensity changes in a real image are rarely clean and sharp changes from one intensity value to another. For one thing, many different changes, slow and fast, often overlap on a variety of different spatial scales. In addition changes in intensity are often corrupted by the visual analogue of noise. They are corrupted, in other words, by random disruptions that infiltrate at different stages as the image formed by the optics of the eye or of a camera is transduced into an array of intensity measurements. In order to cope both with noisy edges and with edges at different spatial scales the image must be "smoothed" by a local averaging of neighboring intensity values. The differencing operation that amounts to the taking of first and second derivatives can then be performed.

There are various ways the sequence can be man-

aged, and much theoretical effort has gone into the search for optimal methods. In one of the simplest the two operations—smoothing and differentiation—are combined into one. In technical terms it sounds forbidding: the image is convolved with a filter that embodies a particular center-surround function, the Laplacian of a Gaussian. It is not as bad as it sounds. A two-dimensional Gaussian is the bell-shaped distribution familiar to statisticians. In this context it specifies the importance to be assigned to the neighborhood of each pixel when the image is being smoothed. As the distance increases, the importance decreases. A Laplacian is a second derivative that gives equal weight to all paths extending away from a point. The Laplacian of a Gaussian converts the bell-shaped distribution into something more like a Mexican hat. The bell is narrowed and at its sides a circular negative dip develops.

Now the procedure can be described nontechnically. Convolving an image with a filter that embodies the Laplacian of a Gaussian is equivalent to substituting for each pixel in the image a weighted average of neighboring pixels, where the weights are provided by the Laplacian of a Gaussian. Thus the filter is applied to each pixel. It assigns the greatest positive weight to that pixel and decreasing positive weights to the pixels nearby (see Figure 5.7). Then comes an annulus—a ring—in

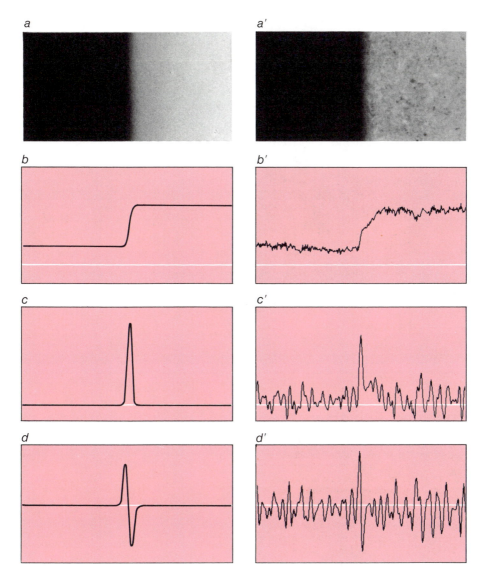

Figure 5.6 SPATIAL DERIVATIVES of an image emphasize its spatial variations in intensity. Left: An edge is
shown between two even shades of gray (*a*). The intensity
along a path across the edge appears below it (*b*). The first
derivative of the intensity is the rate at which intensity
changes (*c*). Toward the left or toward the right there is no
change; the first derivative therefore is zero. Along the
edge itself, however, the rate of change rises and falls. The
second derivative of the intensity is the rate of change of
the rate of change (*d*). Both derivatives emphasize the edge.
The first derivative marks it with a peak; the second derivative marks it by crossing zero. Right: The edge is more
typical of the visual world (*a'*). The related intensity contour (*b'*) and its first and second derivatives (*c'*, *d'*) are
"noisy." The edge must be smoothed before derivatives are
taken.

which the pixels are given negative weightings.
Bright points there feed negative numbers into the
averaging. The result of the overall filtering is an
array of positive and negative numbers: a kind of
second derivative of the image intensity at the scale

of the filter. The zero-crossings in this filtered array
correspond to places in the original image where its
intensity changes most rapidly. Note that a binary
(that is, a two-valued) map showing merely the
positive and negative regions of the filtered array is

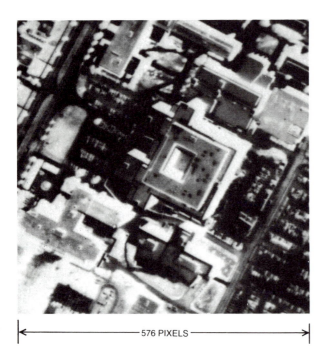

576 PIXELS

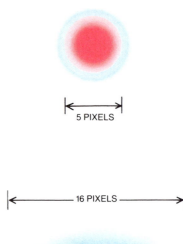

5 PIXELS

16 PIXELS

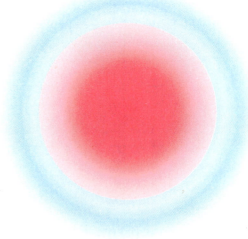

Figure 5.7 CENTER-SURROUND FILTERING of an image serves both to smooth it and to take its second spatial derivative. Left: Image is shown with filters of two sizes depicted schematically; the "filter" is actually computational. Each intensity measurement in the image is replaced by a weighted average of neighboring measurements. Nearby measurements contribute positive weights to the average; thus the filter's center is "excitatory" (*red*). Then comes an annulus, or ring, in which the measurements contribute negative weights; thus the filter's "surround" is "inhibitory" (*blue*). Right: Maps produced by the filters are no longer gray-level arrays. They have both positive values (*red*) and negative values (*blue*). They are maps of the second derivative. Transitions from one color to the other are zero-crossings. The maps emphasize the zero-crossings by showing only positive regions (*red*) and negative regions (*blue*).

essentially equivalent to a map of the zero-crossings in that one can be constructed from the other.

In the human brain most of the hardware required to perform such a filtering seems to be present. As early as 1865 Ernst Mach observed that visual perception seems to enhance spatial varia-

tions in light intensity. He postulated that the enhancement might be achieved by lateral inhibition, a brain mechanism in which the excitation of an axon, or nerve fiber, say by a spot of bright light in the visual world, blocks the excitation of neighboring axons. The operation plainly enhances the con-

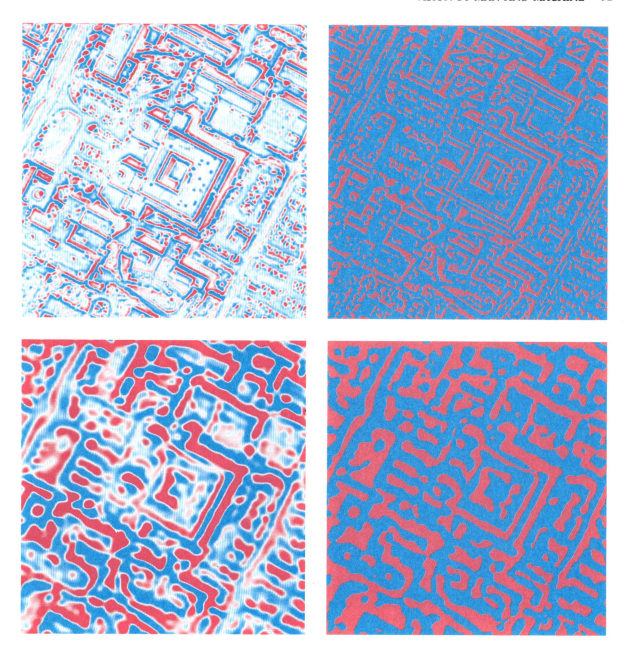

trast between the bright spot and its surroundings. Hence it is similar to the taking of a spatial derivative.

Then in the 1950's and 1960's evidence accumulated suggesting that the retina does something much like center-surround filtering. The output from each retina is conveyed to the rest of the brain by about a million nerve fibers, each being the axon of a neuron called a retinal ganglion cell. The cell derives its input (by way of intermediate neurons) from a group of photoreceptors, which form a "receptive field." What the evidence suggests is that for certain ganglion cells the receptive field has a center-surround organization closely approximating the Laplacian of a Gaussian. Brightness in the center of the receptive field excites the ganglion cell; brightness in a surrounding annulus inhibits it. In short, the receptive field has an ON-center and an OFF-surround, just like the Mexican hat (see Figure 5.8).

Other ganglion cells have the opposite properties: they are OFF-center, ON-surround. If axons could signal negative numbers, these cells would be redundant: they report simply the negation of what the ON-center cells report. Neurons, however, can-

not readily transmit negative activity; the ones that transmit all-or-nothing activity are either active or quiescent. Nature, then, may need neuronal opposites. Positive values in an image subjected to center-surround filtering could be represented by the activity of ON-center cells; negative values could be represented by the activity of OFF-center cells. In this regard I cannot refrain from mentioning the recent finding that ON-center and OFF-center ganglion cells are segregated into two different layers, at least in the retina of the cat. The maps generated

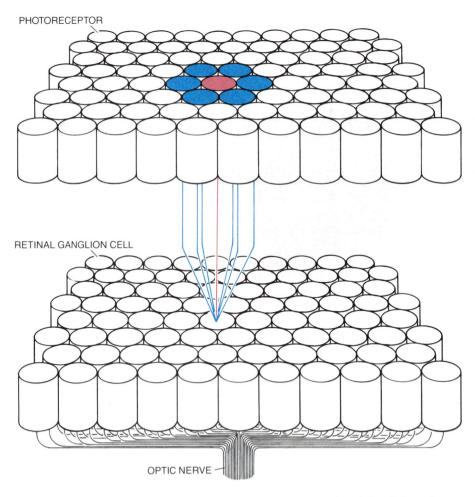

PHOTORECEPTOR

RETINAL GANGLION CELL

OPTIC NERVE

Figure 5.8 BIOLOGICAL CENTER-SURROUND FILTER embodied by cells in the retina resembles the computer procedure shown in Figure 5.7. The filter begins with a layer of photoreceptors connected by way of intermediate nerve cells, not shown in the diagram, to a layer of retinal ganglion cells, which send visual data to higher visual centers. For the sake of simplicity only one set of connections is shown. A photoreceptor cell (*red*) excites an "ON-center" ganglion cell by promoting its tendency to generate neural signals; the surrounding photoreceptors (*blue*) inhibit the ganglion cell.

by our computer might thus depict neural activity rather literally. In the maps in Figure 5.7 red might correspond to ON-layer activity and blue to OFF-layer activity. Zero-crossings (that is, transitions from one color to the other) would be the locations where activity switches from one layer to the other. Here, then, is a conjecture linking a computational theory of vision to the brain hardware serving biological vision.

It should be said that the center-surround filtering of an image is computationally expensive for a computer because it involves great numbers of multiplications: about a billion for an image of 1,000 pixels by 1,000. At the Artificial Intelligence Laboratory, H. Keith Nishihara and Noble G. Larson, Jr., have designed a specialized device: a convolver that performs the operation in about a second. The speed is impressive but is plodding compared with that of the retinal ganglion cells.

I should also mention the issue of spatial scale. In an image there are fine changes in intensity as well as coarse. All must be detected and represented. How can it be done? The natural solution (and the solution suggested by physiology and psychophysics) is to use center-surround filters of different sizes. The filters turn out to be band-pass: they respond optimally to a certain range of spatial frequencies. In other words, they "see" only changes in intensity from pixel to pixel that are neither too fast nor too slow. For any one spatial scale the process of finding intensity changes consists, therefore, of filtering the image with a center-surround filter (or receptive field) of a particular size and then finding the zero-crossings in the filtered image. For a combination of scales it is necessary to set up filters of different sizes, performing the same computation for each scale. Large filters would then detect soft or blurred edges as well as overall illumination changes; small filters would detect finer details. Sharp edges would be detected at all scales.

Recent theoretical results enhance the attractiveness of this idea by showing that features similar to zero-crossings in a filtered image can be rich in information. First, Ben Logan of Bell Laboratories has proved that a one-dimensional signal filtered through a certain class of filters can be reconstructed from its zero-crossings alone. The Laplacian of a Gaussian does not satisfy Logan's conditions exactly. Still, his work suggests that the primitive symbols provided by zero-crossings are potent visual symbols. More recently Alan Yuille

and I have made a theoretical analysis of center-surround filtering. We have been able to show that zero-crossing maps obtained at different scales can represent the original image completely, that is, without any loss of information.

This is not to say that zero-crossings are the optimal coding scheme for a process such as stereopsis. Nor is it to insist that zero-crossings are the sole basis of biological vision. They are a candidate for an optimal coding scheme, and they (or something like them) may be important among the items to be matched between the two retinal images. We have, therefore, a possible answer to the question of what the stereopsis module matches. In addition we have the beginning of a computational theory that may eventually give mathematical precision to the vague concept of "edges" and connect it to known properties of biological vision, such as the prominence of "edge detector" cells discovered at the Harvard Medical School by David H. Hubel and Torsten N. Wiesel in the part of the cerebral cortex where visual data arrive.

To summarize, a combination of computational arguments and biological data suggests that an important first step for stereopsis and other visual processes is the detection and marking of changes in intensity in an image at different spatial scales. One way to do it is to filter the image by the Laplacian of a Gaussian; the zero-crossings in the filtered array will then correspond to intensity edges in the image. Similar information is implicit in the activity of ON-center and OFF-center ganglion cells in the retina. To explicitly represent the zero-crossings (if indeed the brain does it at all) a class of edge-detector neurons in the brain (no doubt in the cerebral cortex) would have to perform specific operations on the output of ON-center and OFF-center cells that are neighbors in the retina. Here, however, one comes up against the lack of information about precisely what elementary computations nerve cells can readily do.

We are now in a position to see how a representation of intensity changes might be useful for stereopsis. Consider first an algorithm devised by Marr and me that implements the constraints discussed above, namely uniqueness (a given point on a physical surface has only one location, so that only one binocular match is correct) and continuity (variations in depth are generally smooth, so that binocular disparities tend to vary smoothly). It is successful at solving random-dot stereograms and at least some natural images. It is done by a computer; thus its actual execution amounts to a sequence of calculations. It can be thought of, however, as setting up a three-dimensional network of nodes, where the nodes represent all possible intersections of lines of sight from the eyes in the three-dimensional world. The uniqueness constraint will then be implemented by requiring that the nodes along a given line of sight inhibit one another. Meanwhile the continuity constraint will be implemented by requiring that each node excite its neighbors. In the case of random-dot stereograms the procedure will be relatively simple. There the matches for pixels on each horizontal row in one stereogram need be sought only along the corresponding row of the other stereogram.

The algorithm starts by assigning a value of 1 to all nodes representing a binocular match between two white pixels or two black pixels in the pair of stereograms. The other nodes are given a value of 0. The 1's thus mark all matches, true and false (see Figure 5.9). Next the algorithm performs an algebraic sum for each node. In it the neighboring nodes with a value of 1 contribute positive weights; the nodes with a value of 1 along lines of sight contribute negative weights. If the result exceeds some threshold value, the node is given the value of 1; otherwise the node is set to 0. That constitutes one iteration of the procedure. After a few such iterations the network reaches stability. The stereopsis problem is solved (see Figure 5-10).

The algorithm has some great virtues. It is a cooperative algorithm: it consists of local calculations that a large number of simple processors could perform asynchronously and in parallel. One imagines that neurons could do them. In addition the algorithm can fill in gaps in the data. That is, it interpolates continuous surfaces. At the same time it allows for sharp discontinuities. On the other hand, the network it would require to process finely detailed natural images would have to be quite large, and most of the nodes in the network would be idle at any one time. Furthermore, intensity values are unsatisfactory for images more natural than random-dot stereograms.

The algorithm's effectiveness can be extended to at least some natural images by first filtering the images to obtain the sign of their convolution with the Laplacian of a Gaussian. The resulting binary maps then serve as inputs for the cooperative algorithm. The maps themselves are intriguing. In the ones generated by large filters at correspondingly low spatial resolution, zero-crossings of a given sign (for instance the crossings at which the sign of the convolution changes from positive to negative) turn out to be quite rare and are never close to each other. Thus false targets (matches between noncorresponding zero-crossings in a pair of stereograms) are essentially absent over a large range of disparities.

This suggests a different class of stereopsis algorithms. One such algorithm, developed recently for robots by Nishihara, matches positive or negative patches in filtered image pairs. Another algorithm, developed earlier by Marr and me, matches zero-crossings of the same sign in image pairs made by filters of three or more sizes. First the coarsely filtered images are matched and the binocular disparities are measured. The results are employed to approximately register the images. (Monocular features such as textures could also be used.) A similar matching process is then applied to the medium-filtered images. Finally the process is applied to the most finely filtered images. By that time the binocular disparities in the stereo pair are known in detail, and so the problem of stereopsis has been reduced to trigonometry.

A theoretical extension and computer implementation of our algorithm by W. Eric L. Grimson at the Artificial Intelligence Laboratory works quite well for a typical application of stereo systems: the analysis of aerial photographs (see Figure 5.1). In addition it mimics many of the properties of human depth perception. For example, it performs successfully when one of the stereo images is out of focus. Yet there may also be subtle differences. Recent work by John Mayhew and John P. Frisby at the University of Sheffield and by Julesz at Bell Laboratories should clarify the matter.

What can one say about biological stereopsis? The algorithms I have described are still far from solving the correspondence problem as effectively as our own brain can. Yet they do suggest how the problem is solved. Meanwhile investigations of the cerebral cortex of the cat and of the cerebral cortex of the macaque monkey have shown that certain cortical neurons signal binocular disparities. And quite recently Gian F. Poggio of the Johns Hopkins University School of Medicine has found cortical neurons that signal the correct binocular disparity in random-dot stereograms in which there are many false matches. His discovery, together with our computational analysis of stereopsis, promises to yield insight into the brain mechanisms underlying depth perception.

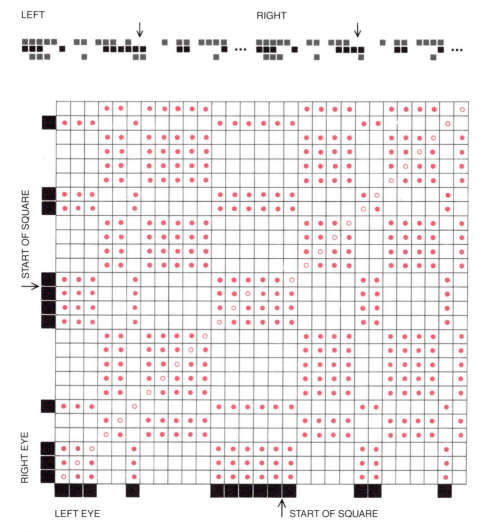

Figure 5.9 STEREOPSIS ALGORITHM reconstructs the three-dimensional visual world by seeking matches between dots on corresponding rows of a pair of random-dot stereograms. Two such rows are shown (*black and white, top*). The rows below are placed along the axes. Horizontal lines represent lines of sight for the right eye; vertical lines, lines of sight for the left. Color marks all intersections at which the eyes both see a black dot or a white dot. A given dot in one stereogram could in principle match any same-color dot in the other. Yet only some matches are correct (*open colored circles*), that is, only some reveal that a square of random-dot texture has a binocular disparity.

One message should emerge clearly: the extent to which the computer and the brain can be brought together for the study of problems such as vision. On the one hand the computer provides a powerful tool for testing computational theories and algorithms. In the process it guides the design of neurophysiological experiments: it suggests what one should look for in the brain. The impetus this will give brain research in the coming decades is likely to be great.

The benefit is not entirely in that direction; computer science also stands to gain. Some computer scientists have maintained that the brain provides only existence proofs, that is, a living demonstration that a given problem has a solution. They are mistaken. The brain can do more: it can show how to seek solutions. The brain is an information processor that has evolved over many millions of years to perform certain tasks superlatively well. If we regard it, with justified modesty, as an uncertain in-

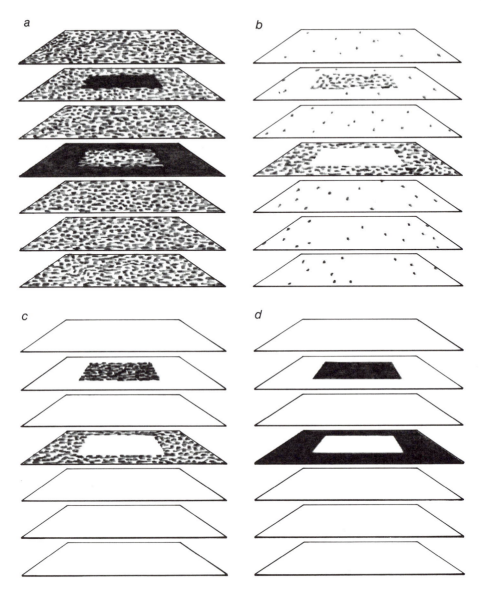

Figure 5.10 ITERATIONS OF THE ALGORITHM (depicted schematically) solve the problem of stereopsis. The algorithm assigns a value of 1 to all intersections of lines of sight marked by a match, and of 0 to the others. Next it calculates a weighted sum for every intersection. Neighboring intersections with a value of 1 contribute positive weights to the sum. The eye sees only one surface along a given line of sight; hence intersections with a value of 1 along lines of sight contribute negative weights. If the result exceeds a threshold value, the intersection is reset to 1; otherwise it is reset to 0. After a few iterations of the procedure the calculation is complete: the stereograms are decoded.

strument, the reason is simply that we tend to be most conscious of the things it does least well—the recent things in evolutionary history, such as logic, mathematics and philosophy—and that we tend to be quite unconscious of its true powers, say in vision. It is in the latter domains that we have much to learn from the brain, and it is in these domains that we should judge our achievements in computer science and in robots. We may then begin to see what vast potential lies ahead.

Features and Objects in Visual Processing

The seemingly effortless ability to perceive meaningful wholes in the visual world depends on complex processes. The features automatically extracted from a scene are assembled into objects.

. . .

Anne Treisman
November, 1986

If you were magically deposited in an unknown city, your first impression would be of recognizable objects organized coherently in a meaningful framework. You would see buildings, people, cars and trees. You would not be aware of detecting colors, edges, movements and distances and of assembling them into multidimensional wholes for which you could retrieve identities and labels from memory. In short, meaningful wholes seem to precede parts and properties, as the Gestalt psychologists emphasized many years ago.

This apparently effortless achievement, which you repeat innumerable times throughout your waking hours, is proving very difficult to understand or to simulate on a computer—much more difficult, in fact, than the understanding and simulation of tasks that most people find quite challenging, such as playing chess or solving problems in logic. The perception of meaningful wholes in the visual world apparently depends on complex operations to which a person has no conscious access, operations that can only be inferred on the basis of indirect evidence (see Figure 6.1).

Nevertheless, some simple generalizations about visual information processing are beginning to emerge. One of them is a distinction between two levels of processing. Certain aspects of visual processing seem to be accomplished simultaneously (that is, for the entire visual field at once) and automatically (that is, without attention being focused on any one part of the visual field). Other aspects of visual processing seem to depend on focused attention and are done serially, or one at a time, as if a mental spotlight were being moved from one location to another.

In 1967 Ulric Neisser, then at the University of Pennsylvania, suggested that a "preattentive" level of visual processing segregates regions of a scene into figures and ground so that a subsequent, attentive level can identify particular objects. More recently David C. Marr, investigating computer simulation of vision at the Massachusetts Institute of Technology, found it necessary to establish a "primal sketch": a first stage of processing, in which the pattern of light reaching an array of receptors in converted into a coded description of lines, spots or edges and their locations, orientations and colors. The representation of surfaces and volumes and finally the identification of objects could begin only after this initial coding.

In brief, a model with two or more stages is gaining acceptance among psychologists, physiologists

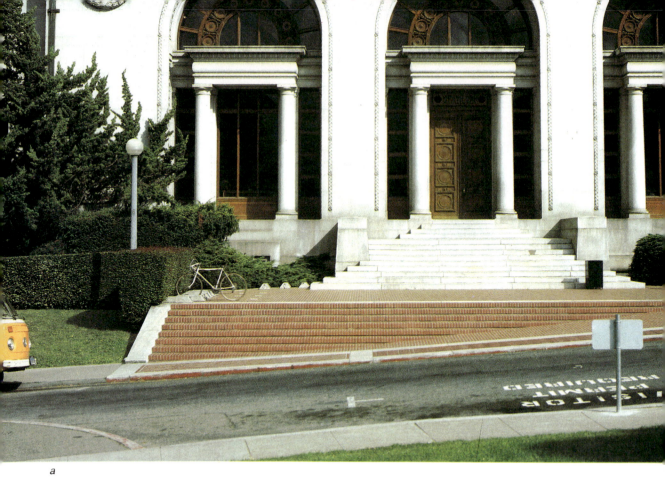

a

Figure 6.1 PRIOR KNOWLEDGE AS A GUIDE in visual perception is tested by asking subjects to search for a familiar object in unjumbled (*a*) and jumbled (*b*) photographs of an unexceptional scene. The task, to find the bicycle, takes longer in the jumbled image because knowledge of the world—about the characteristic locations of bicycles in an urban landscape—speeds up perception and makes it less subject to error. Certain early aspects of the information processing that underlie visual perception nonetheless seem to happen automatically. (Modeled after experiments done by Irving Biederman working at the State University of New York at Buffalo.)

and computer scientists working in artificial intelligence. Its first stage might be described as the extraction of features from patterns of light; later stages are concerned with the identification of objects and their settings. The phrase "features and objects" is therefore a three-word characterization of the emerging hypothesis about the early stages of vision.

I think there are many reasons to agree that vision indeed applies specialized analyzers to decompose stimuli into parts and properties, and that extra operations are needed to specify their recombination into the correct wholes. In part the evidence is physiological and anatomical. In particular, the effort to trace what happens to sensory data suggests that the data are processed in different areas of considerable specialization. One area concerns itself mainly with the orientation of lines and edges, another with color, still another with directions of movement. Only after processing in these areas do data reach areas that appear to discriminate between complex natural objects.

Some further evidence is behavioral. For example, it seems that visual adaptation (the visual system's tendency to become unresponsive to a sustained stimulus) occurs separately for different properties of a scene. If you stare at a waterfall for a few minutes and then look at the bank of the river, the bank will appear to flow in the opposite direction. It is as if the visual detectors had selectively adapted to a particular direction of motion indepen-

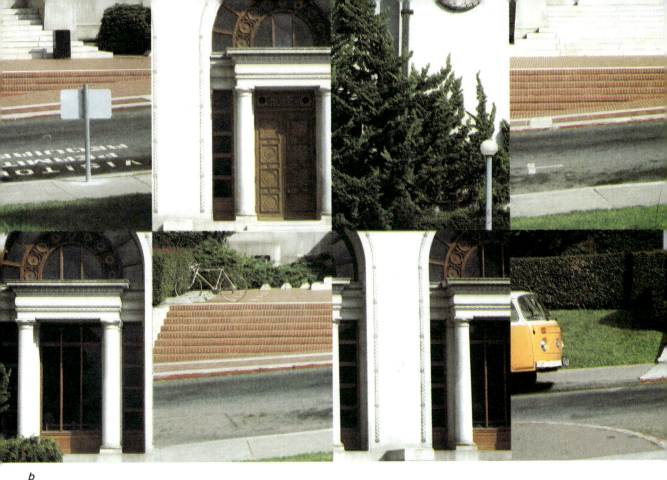

b

dent of *what* is moving. The bank looks very different from the water, but it nonetheless shows the aftereffects of the adaptation process.

How can the preattentive aspect of visual processing be further subjected to laboratory examination? One strategy is suggested by the obvious fact that in the real world parts that belong to the same object tend to share properties: they have the same color and texture, their boundaries show a continuity of lines or curves, they move together, they are at roughly the same distance from the eye. Accordingly the investigator can ask subjects to locate the boundaries between regions in various visual displays and thus can learn what properties make a boundary immediately salient — make it "pop out" of a scene. These properties are likely to be the ones the visual system normally employs in its initial task of segregating figure from ground.

It turns out that boundaries are salient between elements that differ in simple properties such as color, brightness and line orientation but not be-

tween elements that differ in how their properties are combined or arranged (see Figure 6.2). For example, a region of T's segregates well from a region of tilted T's but not from a region of L's made of the same components as the T's (a horizontal line and a vertical line). By the same token, a mixture of blue V's and red O's does not segregate from a mixture of red V's and blue O's. It seems that the early "parsing" of the visual field is mediated by separate properties, not by particular combinations of properties. That is, analysis of properties and parts precedes their synthesis. And if parts or properties are identified before they are conjoined with objects, they must have some independent psychological existence.

This leads to a strong prediction, which is that errors of synthesis should sometimes take place. In other words, subjects should sometimes see illusory conjunctions of parts or properties drawn from different areas of the visual field. In certain condi-

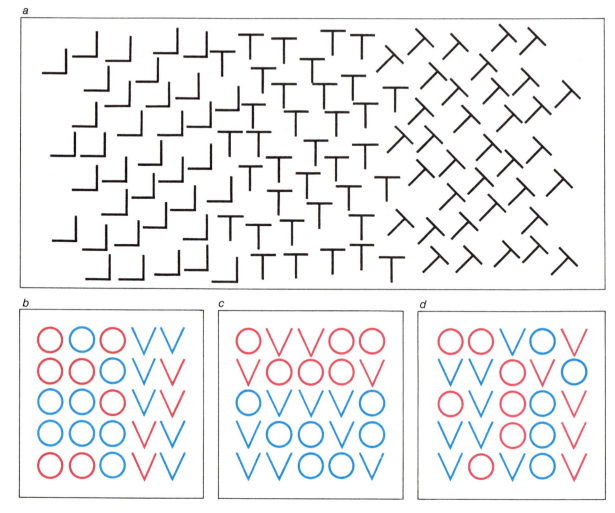

Figure 6.2 EARLY VISION DEALS only with individual features, not with conjunctions of features. A boundary between T's and tilted T's pops out, whereas a boundary between T's and L's does not (*a*). The implication is that line orientations are important features in early visual processing but that particular arrangements of conjunctions of lines are not. A boundary between O's and V's pops out (*b*). The implication is that simple shape properties (such as line curvature) are important. A boundary between red and blue shapes pops out (*c*), implying that color is important. A boundary between conjunctions of shape and color, in this case red V's and blue O's versus red O's and blue V's (*d*), does not pop out.

tions such illusions take place frequently. In one experiment my colleagues and I flashed three colored letters, say a blue X, a green T and a red O, for a brief period (200 milliseconds, or a fifth of a second) and diverted our subjects' attention by asking them to report first a digit shown at each side of the display and only then the colored letters. In about one trial in three the subjects reported the wrong combinations—perhaps a red X, a green O or a blue T.

The subjects made these conjunction errors much more often than they reported a color or shape that was not present in the display, which suggests that the errors reflect genuine exchanges of properties rather than simply misperceptions of a single object. Many of these errors appear to be real illusions, so convincing that subjects demand to see the display again to convince themselves that the errors were indeed mistakes.

We have looked for constraints on the occurrence

of such illusory conjunctions. For example, we have asked whether objects must be similar for their properties to be exchanged. It seems they do not: subjects exchanged colors between a small, red outline of a triangle and a large, solid blue circle just as readily as they exchanged colors between two small outline triangles. It is as if the red color of the triangle were represented by an abstract code for red rather than being incorporated into a kind of analogue of the triangle that also encodes the object's size and shape.

We also asked if it would be harder to create illusory conjunctions by detaching a part from a simple unitary shape, such as a triangle, than by moving a loose line. The answer again was no. Our subjects saw illusory dollar signs in a display of S's and lines. They also saw the illusory signs in a display of S's and triangles in which each triangle incorporated the line the illusion required (see Figure 6.3). In conscious experience the triangle looks like a cohesive whole. Nevertheless, at the preattentive level its component lines seem to be detected independently.

To be sure, the triangle may have an additional feature, namely the fact that its constituent lines enclose an area, and this property of closure might be detected preattentively. If so, the perception of a triangle might require the detection of its three components lines in the correct orientations and also the detection of closure. We should then find that subjects do not see illusory triangles when they are given only the triangles' separate lines in the proper orientations. They may need a further stimulus, a different closed shape (perhaps a circle), in order to assemble illusory triangles. That is indeed what we found (see Figure 6.4).

Another way to make the early, preattentive level of visual processing the subject of laboratory investigation is to assign visual-search tasks. That is, we ask subjects to find a target item in the midst of other, "distractor" items. The assumption is that if the preattentive processing occurs automatically and across the visual field, a target that is distinct from its neighbors in its preattentive representation in the brain should "pop out" of the display. The proverbial needle in a haystack is hard to find because it shares properties of length, thickness and orientation with the hay in which it is hidden. A red poppy in a haystack is a much easier target; its unique color and shape are detected automatically.

We find that if a target differs from the distractors in some simple property, such as orientation or color or curvature, the target is detected about equally fast in an array of 30 items and in an array of three items. Such targets pop out of the display, so that the time it takes to find them is independent of the number of distractors. This independence holds true even when subjects are not told what the unique property of the target will be. The subjects take slightly longer overall, but the number of distractors still has little or no effect.

On the other hand, we find that if a target is characterized only by a conjunction of properties

a

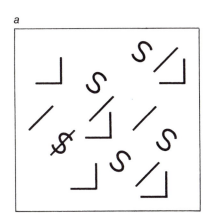

b

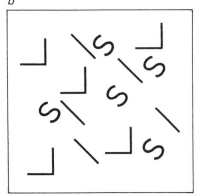

c

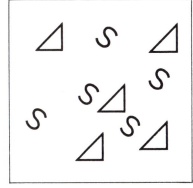

Figure 6.3 ILLUSORY DOLLAR SIGNS are an instance of false conjunctions of features. Subjects were asked to look for dollar signs in the midst of S's and line segments (a). They often reported seeing the signs when the displays to which they were briefly exposed contained none (b). They had the same experience about as often when the line segment needed to complete a sign was embedded in a triangle (c). The experiment suggests that early visual processing can detect the presence of features independent of location.

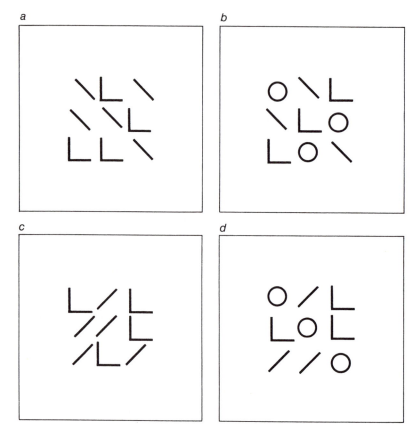

Figure 6.4 ILLUSORY TRIANGLES constitute a test of what features must be available to support the perception of triangles. Subjects seldom reported seeing a triangle when they were briefly exposed to displays consisting of the line segments that make up a triangle (*a*). They saw triangles far more often when the displays also included closed stimuli, that is, shapes that enclose a space, in this case O's (*b*). Evidently closure is a feature analyzed in early visual processing. This conclusion was supported by showing displays that lack the diagonal line to make a triangle (*c, d*). Subjects seldom saw triangles in such displays.

(for example, a red O among red N's and green O's) (see Figure 6.5), or if it is defined only by its particular combination of components (for example, an R among P's and Q's that together incorporate all the parts of the R), the time taken to find the target or to decide that the target is not present increases linearly with the number of distractors. It is as if the subjects who are placed in these circumstances are forced to focus attention in turn on each item in the display in order to determine how the item's properties or parts are conjoined. In a positive trial (a trial in which a target is present) the search ends when the target is found; on the average, therefore, it ends after half of the distractors have been exam-

ined. In a negative trial (in which no target is present) all the distractors have to be checked. As distractors are added to the displays, the search time in positive trials therefore increases at half the rate of the search time in negative trials.

The difference between a search for simple features and a search for conjunctions of features could have implications in industrial settings. Quality-control inspectors might, for example, take more time to check manufactured items if the possible errors in manufacture are characterized by faulty combinations of properties than they do if the errors always result in a salient change in a single property. Similarly, each of the symbols representing,

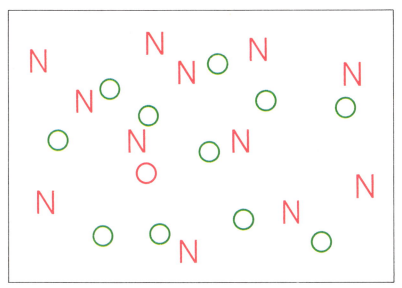
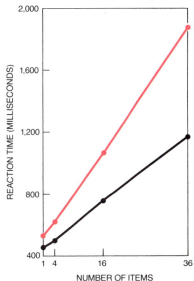

Figure 6.5 "DISTRACTOR ITEMS" LENGTHEN the search for a target item defined by a conjunction of features. Here the target is a red O; the distractors are green O's and red N's. When no target was present, the average search time increased by some 40 milliseconds for each distractor added to the display; when a target was present (so that subjects had to search half the items before finding the target), the search time increased at roughly half that rate. A target characterized by a conjunction of properties requires subjects to focus attention on each displayed item in turn. If a target has a unique color or shape, the number of distractors does not influence search time.

say, the destinations for baggage handled at airline terminals should be characterized by a unique combination of properties.

In a further series of experiments on visual-search tasks, we explored the effect of exchanging the target and the distractors. That is, we required subjects to find a target distinguished by the fact that it *lacks* a feature present in all the distractors. For example, we employed displays consisting of O's and Q's, so that the difference between the target and the distractors is that one is simply a circle whereas the other is a circle intersected by a line segment (see Figure 6.6). We found a remarkable difference in the search time depending on whether the target was the Q and had the line or was the O and lacked the line. When the target had the line, the search time was independent of the number of distractors. Evidently the target popped out of the display. When the target lacked the line, the search time increased linearly with the number of distractors. Evidently, the items in the display were being subjected to a serial search.

The result goes against one's intuitions. After all, each case involves the same discrimination between the same two stimuli: O's and Q's. The result is consistent, however, with the idea that a pooled neural signal early in visual processing conveys the presence but not the absence of a distinctive feature. In other words, early vision extracts simple properties, and each type of property triggers activity in populations of specialized detectors. A target with a unique property is detected in the midst of distractor items simply by a check on whether the relevant detectors are active. Conversely, a target lacking a property that is present in the distractors arouses only slightly less activity than a display consisting exclusively of distractors. We propose, therefore, that early vision sets up a number of what might be called feature maps. They are not necessarily to be equated with the specialized visual areas that are mapped by physiologists, although the correspondence is suggestive.

We have exploited visual-search tasks to test a wide range of candidate features we thought might pop out of displays and so reveal themselves as primitives: basic elements in the language of early vision. The candidates fell into a number of catego-

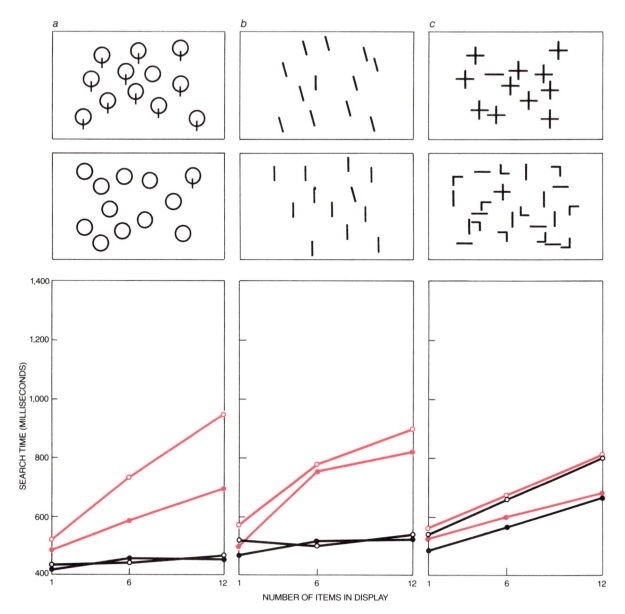

Figure 6.6 PRESENCE OR ABSENCE of a feature affects the time it takes to find a target in the midst of distractors. In one experiments (*a*) the target was a circle intersected by a vertical line segment or a circle without that feature. The search time for the intersected circle (*black*) was largely independent of the number of items in the display, suggesting that the feature popped out. The search time for the plain circle (*color*) increased steeply as distractors were added, suggesting that a serial search of the display was

ries: quantitative properties such as length or number; properties of single lines such as orientation or curvature; properties of line arrangements; topological and relational properties such as the connectedness of lines, the presence of the free ends of lines or the ratio of the height to the width of a shape.

Among the quantitative candidates, my colleagues and I found that some targets popped out when their discriminability was great. In particular, the more extreme targets—the longer lines, the darker grays, the pairs of lines (when the distractors were single lines)—were easier to detect. This sug-

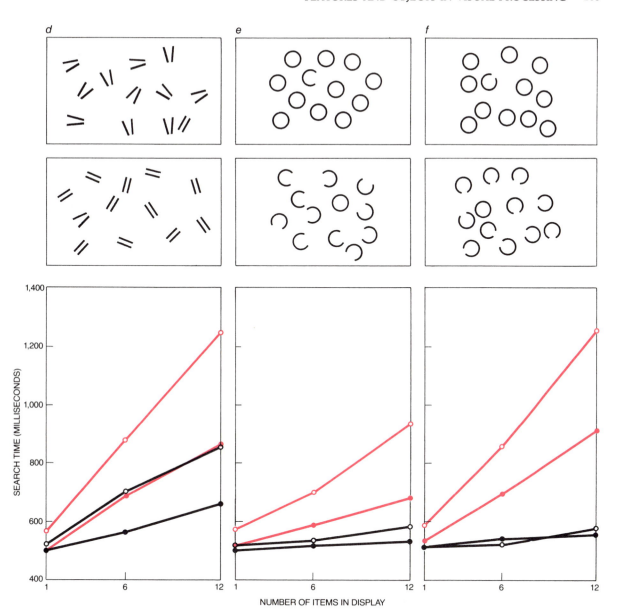

being made. Other experiments compared (b) the search times for a vertical (*color*) or a tilted line (*black*); (c) an isolated line segment (*color*) or an intersection of lines, a plus (*black*); (d) parallel lines (*color*) or converging lines (*black*); (e) closure using complete circles (*color*) or circles with a gap (*black*); (f) closure again using complete circles (*color*) or circles with smaller gaps (*black*). Open dots show data from trials in which display had only distractors.

gests that the visual system responds positively to "more" in these quantitative properties and that "less" is coded by default. For example, the neural activity signaling line length might increase with increasing length (up to some maximum), so that a longer target is detected against the lower level of background activity produced by short distractors. In contrast, a shorter target, with its concomitant lower rate of firing, is likely to be swamped by the greater activity produced by the longer distractors. Psychophysicists have known for more than a century that the ability to distinguish differences in intensity grows more acute with decreasing background intensity. We suggest that the same phenomenon, which is known as Weber's law, could account for our findings concerning the quantitative features.

Our tests of two simple properties of lines, orientation and curvature, yielded some surprises. In both cases we found pop-out for one target, a tilted line among vertical distractors (see Figure 6.6*b*) and a curved line among straight lines, but not for the converse target, a vertical line among tilted distractors and a straight line among curves. These findings suggest that early vision encodes tilt and curvature but not verticality or straightness. That is, the vertical targets and the straight targets appear to lack a feature the distractors possess, as if they represent null values on their respective dimensions. If our interpretation is correct, it implies that in early vision tilt and curvature are represented relationally, as deviations from a standard or norm that itself is not positively signaled.

A similar conclusion emerged for the property of closure. We asked subjects to search for complete circles in the midst of circles with gaps and for circles with gaps among complete circles. Again we found a striking asymmetry, this time suggesting that the gap is preattentively detectable but that closure is not—or rather that it becomes preattentively detectable only when the distractors have very large gaps (that is, when they are quite open shapes like semicircles). In other words, closure is preattentively detectable, but only when the distractors do not share it to any significant degree. On the other hand, gaps (or the line ends that gaps create) are found equally easily whatever their size (unless they are too small for a subject, employing peripheral vision, to see). (See Figure 6.6*e* and *f*.)

Finally, we found no evidence that any property of line arrangements is preattentively detectable. We tested intersections, junctions, convergent lines and parallel lines. In every case we found that search time increases with an increasing number of distractors. The targets become salient and obvious only when the subject's attention is directed to them; they do not emerge automatically when that attention is disseminated throughout the display. (See Figure 6.6*c* and *d*.)

In sum, it seems that only a small number of features are extracted early in visual processing. They include color, size, contrast, tilt, curvature and line ends. Research by other investigators shows that movement and differences in stereoscopic depth are also extracted automatically in early vision. In general the building blocks of vision appear to be simple properties that characterize local elements, such as points or lines, but not the relations among them. Closure appears to be the most complex property that pops out preattentively. Finally, our findings suggest that several preattentive properties are coded as values of deviation from a null, or reference, value.

Up to this point I have concentrated on the initial, preattentive stages of vision. I turn now to the later stages. In particular I turn to the evidence that focused attention is required for conjoining the features at a given location in a scene and for establishing structured representations of objects and their relations.

One line of evidence suggesting that conjunctions require attention emerges from experiments in which we asked subjects to identify a target in a display and say where it was positioned. In one type of display only a simple feature distinguished the target from the distractors. For example, the target was a red H in the midst of red O's and blue X's or an orange X among red O's and blue X's. In other displays the target differed only in the way its features were conjoined. For example, it was a blue O or a red X among red O's and blue X's.

We were particularly interested in the cases in which a subject identified the target correctly but gave it the wrong location. As we expected, the subjects could sometimes identify a simple target, say a target distinguished merely by its color, but get its location wrong. Conjunction targets were different: the correct identification was completely dependent on the correct localization. It does indeed seem that attention must be focused on a location in order to combine the features it contains.

In a natural scene, of course, many conjunctions of features are ruled out by prior knowledge. You seldom come across blue bananas or furry eggs. Preattentive visual processing might be called "bottom up," in that it happens automatically, without any recourse to such knowledge. Specifically, it happens without recourse to "top down" constraints. One might hypothesize that conjunction illusions in everyday life are prevented when they conflict with top-down expectations. There are many demonstrations that we do use our knowledge of the world to speed up perception and to make it more accurate. For example, Irving Biederman working at the State University of New York at Buffalo (now at the University of Minnesota) asked subjects to find a target object such as a bicycle in a photograph of a natural scene or in a jumbled image in which different areas had been randomly interchanged. The subjects did better when the bicycle could be found in a natural context (see Figure 6.1).

In order to explore the role of prior knowledge in the conjoining of properties, Deborah Butler and I did a further study of illusory conjunctions. We showed subjects a set of three colored objects flanked on each side by a digit (see Figure 6.7). Then, some 200 milliseconds later, we showed them a pointer, which was accompanied by a random checkerboard in order to wipe out any visual persistence from the initial display. We asked the subjects to attend to the two digits and report them, and then to say which object the pointer had designated. The sequence was too brief to allow the subjects to focus their attention on all three objects.

The crucial aspect of the experiment lay in the

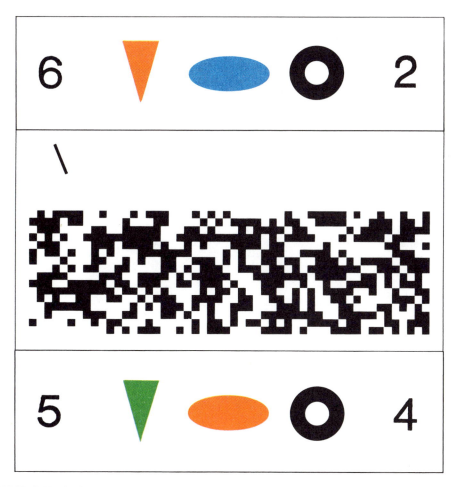

Figure 6.7 EFFECT OF EXPECTATIONS on the perception of conjunctions of features is complex. Subjects were shown three colored shapes flanked on each side by a distractor, specifically a digit (*top*). The display was followed by a masking field and a pointer (*middle*) indicating the prior location of the shape the subject was called on to report. The subjects made many mistakes in associating colors with shapes when they expected arbitrary pairings of colors and shapes (an orange triangle, a blue ellipse and a black ring) but made fewer mistakes when they were expecting pictures of familiar objects (a carrot, a lake and a tire). Surprisingly, when the display showed unexpected combinations instead of natural ones (*bottom*), subjects were not likely to recombine the objects and colors to fit expectation.

labels we gave the objects. We told one group of subjects that the display would consist of "an orange carrot, a blue lake and a black tire." Occasional objects (one in four) were shown in the wrong color to ensure that the subjects could not just name the color they would know in advance ought to be associated with a given shape. For another group of subjects the same display was described as "an orange triangle, a blue ellipse and a black ring."

The results were significant. The group given arbitrary pairings of colors and shapes reported many illusory conjunctions: 29 percent of all their responses represented illusory recombinations of colors and shapes from the display, whereas 13 percent were reports of colors or shapes not present in the display. In contrast, the group expecting familiar objects saw rather few illusory conjunctions: they wrongly recombined colors and shapes only 5 percent more often than they reported colors and shapes not present in the display.

We occasionally gave a third group of subjects the wrong combinations when they were expecting most objects to be in their natural colors (see Figure 6.7, bottom). To our surprise we found no evidence that subjects generated illusory conjunctions to fit their expectations. For example, they were no more likely to see the triangle (the "carrot") as orange when another object in the display was orange than they were when no orange was present. There seem to be two implications: prior knowledge and expec-

tations do indeed help one to use attention efficiently in conjoining features, but prior knowledge and expectations seem not to induce illusory exchanges of features to make abnormal objects normal again. Thus illusory conjunctions seem to arise at a stage of visual processing that precedes semantic access to knowledge of familiar objects. The conjunctions seem to be generated preattentively from the sensory data, bottom-up, and not to be influenced by top-down constraints.

How are objects perceived once attention has been focused on them and the correct set of properties has been selected from those present in the scene? In particular, how does one generate and maintain an object's perceptual unity even when objects move and change? Imagine a bird perched on a branch, seen from a particular angle and in a particular illumination. Now watch its shape, its size and its color all change as it preens itself, opens its wings and flies away. In spite of these major transformations in virtually all its properties, the bird retains its perceptual integrity: it remains the same single object.

Daniel Kahneman of the University of California at Berkeley and I have suggested that object perception is mediated not only by recognition, or matching to a stored label or description, but also by the construction of a temporary representation that is specific to the object's current appearance and is

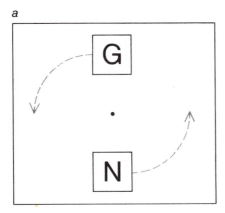

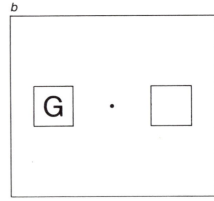

Figure 6.8 INTEGRATION OF SENSORY INFORMATION into a file on each object was tested by the motion of frames. Two frames appeared; then two letters were briefly flashed in the frames (a). The frames moved to new locations, and a letter appeared in one of the two (b). The task was to name the final letter as quickly as possible. If the final letter matched the initial letter and appeared in the same frame, the naming was faster than if the letter had appeared in the other frame or differed from the initial letter, presumably because it takes more time to create or update a file on an object than to perceive the object a second time.

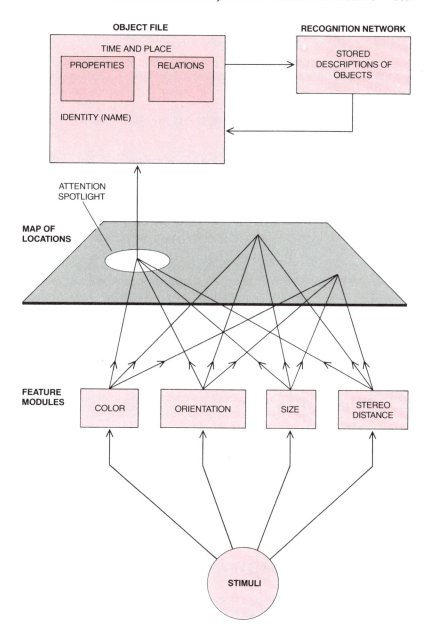

Figure 6.9 HYPOTHETICAL MODEL proposes that early vision encodes some simple and useful properties of a scene in a number of feature maps, which may preserve the spatial relations of the visual world but do not themselves make spatial information available to subsequent processing stages. Instead focused attention (with a master map of locations) selects and integrates features at particular locations. At later stages the integrated information creates and updates files on perceptual objects. The file contents are compared with descriptions stored in a recognition network that incorporates the attributes of familiar objects.

constantly updated as the object changes. We have drawn an analogy to a file in which all the perceptual information about a particular object is entered, just as the police might open a file on a particular crime, in which they collect all the information about the crime as the information accrues. The perceptual continuity of an object would then depend on its current manifestation being allocated to the same file as its earlier appearances. Such allocation is possible if the object remains stationary or if it changes location within constraints that allow the perceptual system to keep track of which file it should belong to.

In order to test this idea we joined with Brian Gibbs in devising a letter-naming task (see Figure 6.8). Two letters were briefly flashed in the centers of two frames. The empty frames then moved to new locations. Next another letter appeared in one of the two frames. We devised the display so that the temporal and spatial separations between the priming letter and the final letter were always the same; the only thing that differed was the motion of the frames. The subjects' task was to name the final letter as quickly as possible.

We knew that the prior exposure to a given letter should normally lessen the time it takes to identify the same letter on a subsequent appearance; the effect is known as priming. The question that interested us was whether priming would occur only in particular circumstances. We argued that if the final letter is the same as the priming letter and appears in the same frame as the priming letter, the two should be seen as belonging to the same object; in this case we could think of the perceptual task as simply re-viewing the original object in its shifted position. If, on the other hand, a new letter appears in the same frame, the object file should have to be updated, perhaps increasing the time it takes for subjects to become aware of the letter and name it.

Actually the priming was found to be object-specific: subjects named the final letter some 30 milliseconds faster if the same letter had appeared previously in the same frame. They showed no such benefit if the same letter had appeared previously in the other frame. The result is consistent with the hypothesis that the later stages of visual perception integrate information from the early, feature-sensitive stages in temporary object-specific representations.

The overall scheme I propose for visual processing can be put in the form of a model (see Figure 6.9). The visual system begins by coding a certain number of simple and useful properties in what can be considered a stack of maps. In the brain such maps ordinarily preserve the spatial relations of the visual world itself. Nevertheless, the spatial information they contain may not be directly available to the subsequent stages of visual processing. Instead the presence of each feature may be signaled without a specification of *where* it is.

In the subsequent stages focused attention acts. In particular, focused attention is taken to operate by means of a master map of locations, in which the presence of discontinuities in intensity or color is registered without specification of what the discontinuities are. Attention makes use of this master map, simultaneously selecting, by means of links to the separate feature maps, all the features that currently are present in a selected location. These are entered into a temporary object representation, or file.

Finally, the model posits that the integrated information about the properties and structural relations in each object file is compared with stored descriptions in a "recognition network." The network specifies the critical attributes of cats, trees, bacon and eggs, one's grandmothers and all the other familiar perceptual objects, allowing access to their names, their likely behavior and their current significance. I assume that conscious awareness depends on the object files and on the information they contain. It depends, in other words, on representations that collect information about particular objects, both from the analyses of sensory features and from the recognition network, and continually update the information. If a significant discontinuity in space or time occurs, the original file on an object may be canceled: it ceases to be a source of perceptual experience. As for the object, it disappears and is replaced by a new object with its own new temporary file, ready to begin a new perceptual history.

OBJECT AND EVENT PERCEPTION

. . .

The Perception of Disoriented Figures

Many familiar things do not look the same when their orientation is changed. The reason appears to be that the perception of form embodies the automatic assignment of a top, a bottom and sides.

. . .

Irvin Rock
January, 1974

Many common experiences of everyday life that we take for granted present challenging scientific problems. In the field of visual perception one such problem is why things look different when they are upside down or tilted. Consider the inverted photograph in Figure 7.1. Although the face is familiar to most Americans, it is difficult to recognize when it is inverted. Even when one succeeds in identifying the face, it continues to look strange and the specific facial expression is hard to make out.

Consider also what happens when printed words and words written in longhand are turned upside down. With effort the printed words can be read, but it is all but impossible to read the longhand words (see Figure 7.2). Try it with a sample of your own handwriting. One obvious explanation of why it is hard to read inverted words is that we have acquired the habit of moving our eyes from left to right, and that when we look at inverted words our eyes tend to move in the wrong direction. This may be one source of the difficulty, but it can hardly be the major one. It is just as hard to read even a single inverted word when we look at it without moving our eyes at all. It is probable that the same factor

interfering with the recognition of disoriented faces and other figures is also interfering with word recognition.

The partial rotation of even a simple figure can also prevent its recognition, provided that the observer is unaware of the rotation. A familiar figure viewed in a novel orientation no longer appears to have the same shape (see Figure 7.3). As Ernst Mach pointed out late in the 19th century, the appearance of a square is quite different when it is rotated 45 degrees. In fact, we call it a diamond (see Figure 7.4).

Some may protest that a familiar shape looks different in a novel orientation for the simple reason that we rarely see it that way. But even a figure we have not seen before will look different in different orientations (see Figure 7.5). The fact is that orientation affects perceived shape, and that the failure to recognize a familiar figure when it is in a novel orientation is based on the change in its perceived shape.

On the other hand, a figure can be changed in various ways without any effect on its perceived shape. For example, a triangle can be altered in size, color and various other ways without any change in

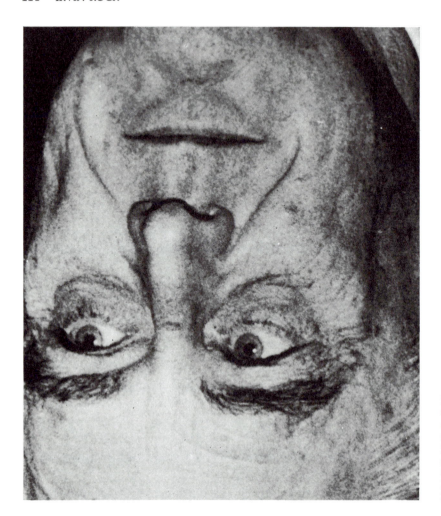

Figure 7.1 INVERTED PHOTO-GRAPH of a famous American demonstrates how difficult it is to recognize a familiar face when it is presented upside down. Even after one succeeds in identifying the inverted face as that of Frank-lin D. Roosevelt, it continues to look strange.

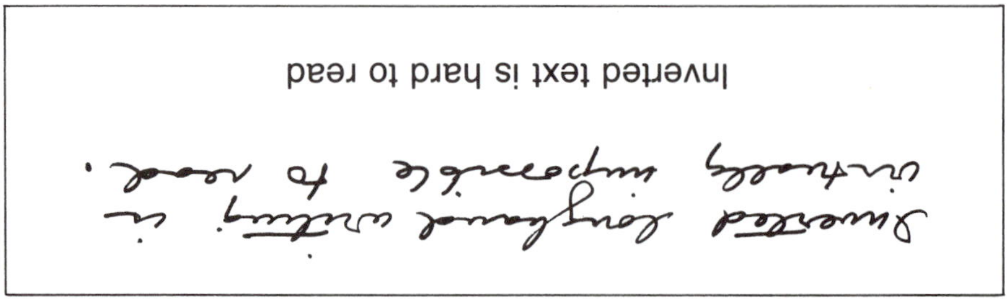

Inverted text is hard to read

Figure 7.2 INVERTED WORDS are difficult to read when they are set in type, and words written in longhand are virtually impossible to decipher. The difficulty applies to one's own inverted handwriting in spite of a lifetime of experience reading it in the normal upright orientation.

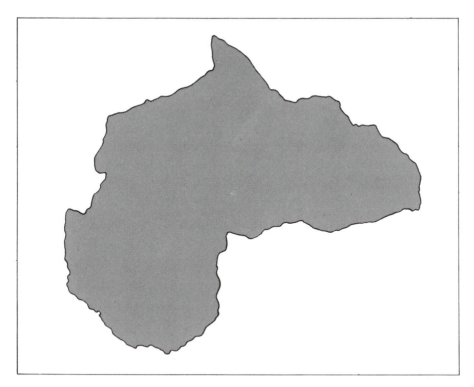

Figure 7.3 "UNFAMILIAR" SHAPE shown here becomes a familiar shape when it is rotated clockwise 90 degrees. In a classroom experiment, when the rotated figure was drawn on the blackboard, it was not recognized as an outline of the continent of Africa until the teacher told the class at the end of the lecture that the figure was rotated out of its customary orientation.

its perceived shape (see Figure 7.6). Psychologists, drawing an analogy with a similar phenomenon in music, call such changes transpositions. A melody can be transposed to a new key, and although all the notes then are different, there is no change in the melody. In fact, we generally remain unaware of the transposition. Clearly the melody derives from the relation of the notes to one another, which is not altered when the melody is transposed. In much the same way a visual form is based primarily on how parts of a figure are related to one another geometrically. For example, one could describe a

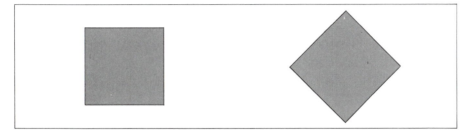

Figure 7.4 SQUARE AND DIAMOND are two familiar shapes. The two figures shown here are identical; their appearance is so different, however, that we call one a square and the other a diamond. With the diamond the angles do not spontaneously appear as right angles.

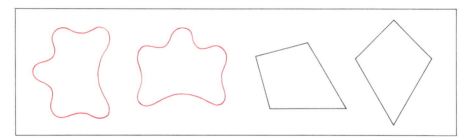

Figure 7.5 NOVEL OR UNFAMILIAR FIGURES look different in different orientations (provided that we view them naïvely and do not mentally rotate them) because of the way a figure is "described" by the perceptual system. The colored figure (*left*) could be described as a closed shape on a horizontal base with a protrusion on its left side and an indentation on its right side; the colored figure adjacent to it as a symmetrical shape resting on a curved base with a protrusion at the top. The first black figure could be described as a quadrilateral resting on a side; the second black figure as a diamondlike shape standing on end.

square as being a four-sided figure having parallel opposite sides, four right angles and four sides of equal length. These features remain unchanged when a square is transposed in size or position; that is why it continues to look like a square. We owe a debt to the Gestalt psychologists for emphasizing the importance in perception of relations rather than absolute features.

Since a transposition based on rotation does not alter the internal geometric relations of a figure, then why does it look different in an altered orientation? At this point we should consider the meaning of the term orientation. What changes are introduced by altering orientation? One obvious change is that rotating a figure would result in a change in the orientation of its image on the retina of the eye. Perhaps, therefore, we should ask why different retinal orientations of the same figure should give rise to different perceived shapes. That might lead us into speculations about how the brain processes information about form, and why differently oriented projections of a retinal image should lead to different percepts of form.

Before we go further in this direction we should consider another meaning of the term orientation. The inverted and rotated figures in the illustrations for this article are in different orientations with

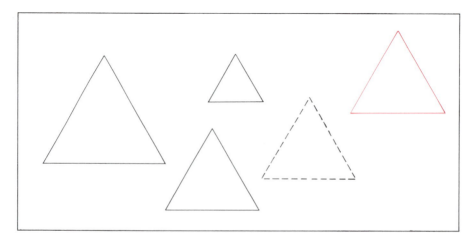

Figure 7.6 ALTERATION IN SIZE, color or type of contour does not change the perceived shape of a triangle. Even varying the location of the triangle's retinal image (by looking out of the corner of your eyes or fixating on different points) does not change perceived shape.

respect to the vertical and horizontal directions in their environment. That part of the figure which is normally pointed upward in relation to gravity, to the sky or to the ceiling, is now pointed downward or sideways on the page. Perhaps it is this kind of orientation that is responsible for altered perception of shape when a figure is disoriented.

It is not difficult to separate the retinal and the environmental factors in an experiment. Cut out a paper square and tape it to the wall so that the bottom of the square is parallel to the floor. Compare the appearance of the square first with your head upright and then with your head tilted 45 degrees. You will see that the square continues to look like a square when your head is tilted. Yet when your head is tilted 45 degrees, the retinal image of the square is the same as the image of a diamond when the diamond is viewed with the head upright. Thus it is not the retinal image that is responsible for the altered appearance of a square when the square is rotated 45 degrees. The converse experiment points to the same conclusion. Rotate the square on the wall so that it becomes a diamond. The diamond viewed with your head tilted 45 degrees produces a retinal image of a square, but the diamond still looks like a diamond. Needless to say, in these simple demonstrations one continues to perceive correctly where the top, bottom and sides of the figures are even when one's posture changes. It is therefore the change of a figure's perceived orientation in the environment that affects its apparent shape and not the change of orientation of its retinal image.

These conclusions have been substantiated in experiments Walter I. Heimer and I and other colleagues have conducted with numerous subjects. In one series of experiments the subjects were shown unfamiliar figures. In the first part of the experiment a subject sat at a table and simply looked at several figures shown briefly in succession. Then some of the subjects were asked to tilt their head 90 degrees by turning it to the side and resting it on the table. In this position the subject viewed a series of figures. Most of the figures were new, but among them were some figures the subject had seen earlier. These figures were shown in either of two orientations: upright with respect to the room (as they had been in the first viewing) or rotated 90 degrees so that the "top" of the figure corresponded to the top of the subject's tilted head. The subject was asked to say whether or not he had seen each figure in the first session. He did not know that the orientation of

the figures seen previously might be different. Other subjects viewed the test figures while sitting upright. (See Figure 7.7.)

When we compared the scores of subjects who tilted their head with subjects who sat upright for the test, the results were clear. Tilted-head subjects recognized the environmentally upright (but retinally tilted) figures about as well as the upright observers did. They also failed to recognize the environmentally tilted (but retinally upright) figures about as often as the upright subjects did. In other words, the experiments confirmed that it is rotation with respect to the up-down and left-right coordinates in the environment that produces the change in the perceived shape of the figure. It is not rotation of the retinal image that produces the change, since altering the image's orientation does not adversely affect recognition and preserving it does not improve recognition.

In another experiment subjects viewed an ambiguous or reversible figure that could be perceived in one of two ways depending on its orientation. For example, when one figure that looked like a map of the U.S. was rotated 90 degrees, it looked like the profile of a bearded man. Subjects were asked to rest their head on the table when viewing the ambiguous figures. The question we asked ourselves was: Which "upright" would dominate, the retinal upright or the environmental upright? The results were decisive. About 80 percent of the subjects reported seeing only the aspect of the ambiguous figure that was environmentally upright, even though the alternative was upright on their retina. (See Figure 7.8.)

Why does the orientation of a figure with respect to the directional coordinates of the environment have such a profound effect on the perceived shape of the figure? The answer I propose is that perceived shape is based on a cognitive process in which the characteristics of the figure are implicitly described by the perceptual system. For example, the colored figure at the left in Figure 7.5 could be described as a closed figure resting on a horizontal base with a protrusion on the figure's left side and an indentation on its right side. The colored figure to the right of it, although it is identical and only rotated 90 degrees, would be described quite differently, as being symmetrical with two bumps on the bottom and with left and right sides more or less straight and identical with each other. I am not suggesting that such a description is conscious or

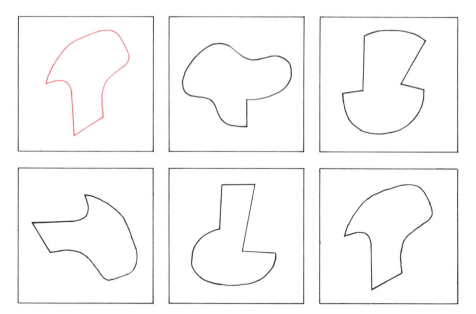

Figure 7.7 ROTATION OF RETINAL IMAGE by tilting the head does not appreciably affect recognition of a novel figure (*color*). Subjects first viewed several novel targets while sitting upright. Then they were shown a series of test figures (*black*) and were asked to identify those they had seen before. Subjects who tilted their heads 90 degrees failed to recognize figures that were retinally "upright" (for example, figure at bottom left) about as much as upright viewers did (to whom such figures were not retinally "upright"). Tilted-head subjects recognized environmentally upright figures (*bottom right*) as often as upright viewers did.

verbal; obviously we would be aware of the descriptive process if it were either. Furthermore, animals and infants who are nonverbal perceive shape much as we do. I am proposing that a process analogous to such a description does take place and that it is not only based on the internal geometry of a figure but takes into account the location of the figure's top, bottom and sides. In such a description orientation is therefore a major factor in the shape that is finally perceived.

From experiments I have done in collaboration with Phyllis Olshansky it appears that certain shifts in orientation have a marked effect on perceived shape. In particular, creating symmetry around a vertical axis where no symmetry had existed before (or vice versa), shifting the long axis from vertical to horizontal (or vice versa) and changing the bottom of a figure from a broad horizontal base to a pointed angle (or vice versa) seemed to have a strong effect on perceived shape. Such changes of shape can result from only a moderate angular change of orientation, say 45 or 90 degrees. Interestingly enough, inversions or rotations of 180 degrees often have only a slight effect on perceived shape, perhaps because such changes will usually not alter per-

ceived symmetry or the perceived orientation of the long axis of the figure.

There is one kind of orientation change that has virtually no effect on perceived shape: a mirror-image reversal. This is particularly true for the novel figures we used in our experiments. How can this be explained? It seems that although the "sides" of visual space are essentially interchangeable, the up-and-down directions in the environment are not. "Up" and "down" are distinctly different directions in the world we live in. Thus a figure can be said to have three main perceptual boundaries: top, bottom and sides. As a result the description of a figure will not be much affected by whether a certain feature is on the left side or the right. Young children and animals have great difficulty learning to discriminate between a figure and its mirror image, but they can easily distinguish between a figure and its inverted counterpart.

Related to this analysis is a fact observed by Mach and tested by Erich Goldmeier: a figure that is symmetrical around one axis will generally appear to be symmetrical only if that axis is vertical (see Figure 7.9). Robin Leaman and I have demonstrated that it is the perceived vertical axis of the figure and not

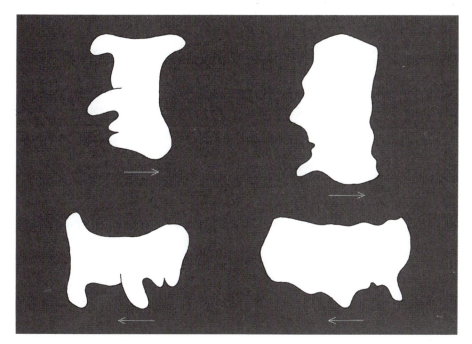

Figure 7.8 AMBIGUOUS FIGURES can be perceived in different ways depending on the orientation assigned to them. Figure at left can look like the profile of a man's head with a chef's hat (*top left*) or, when rotated 90 degrees, like a dog (*bottom left*). Figure at right can look like the profile of a bearded man's head (*top right*) or like a map of the U.S. (*bottom right*). When subjects with their head tilted 90 degrees to one side viewed these ambiguous figures (*direction of subject's head is shown by arrow*), they preferentially recognized the figure that was upright in the environment instead of the figure that was upright on the retina.

the vertical axis of the figure's retinal image that produces this effect. An observer who tilts his head will continue to perceive a figure as being symmetrical if that figure is symmetrical around an environmental vertical axis. This suggests that perceived asymmetry results only when the two equivalent halves of a figure are located on the two equivalent sides of perceptual space.

If, as I have suggested, the description of a figure is based on the location of its top, bottom and sides,

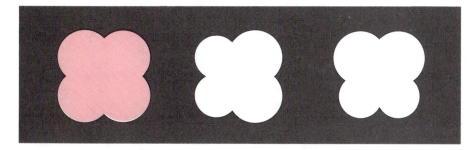

Figure 7.9 IMPRESSION OF SYMMETRY is spontaneous only when a figure is symmetrical around a vertical axis. Subjects asked to indicate which of two figures (*middle and right*) was most like the target figure (*left*) selected the figure at right most frequently, presumably because it is symmetrical around its vertical axis. If the page is tilted 90 degrees, the figure in the middle will now be selected as being more similar to the target figure. Now if the page is held vertically and the figures are viewed with the head tilted 45 degrees, the figure at right is likely to be seen as being the most similar.

the question arises: How are these directions assigned in a figure? One might suppose that the top of a figure is ordinarily the area uppermost in relation to the ceiling, the sky or the top of a page. In a dark room an observer may have to rely on his sense of gravity to inform him which way is up.

Numerous experiments by psychologists have confirmed that there are indeed two major sources of information for perceiving the vertical and the horizontal: gravity (as it is sensed by the vestibular apparatus in the inner ear, by the pressure of the ground on the body and by feedback from the muscles) and information from the scene itself. We have been able to demonstrate that either can affect the perceived shape of a figure. A luminous figure in a dark room will not be recognized readily when it is rotated to a new orientation even if the observer is tilted by exactly the same amount. Here the only source of information about directions in space is gravity. In a lighted room an observer will often fail to recognize a figure when he and the figure are upright but the room is tilted. The tilted room creates a strong impression of where the up-down axis should be, and this leads to an incorrect attribution of the top and bottom of the figure [see "The Perception of the Upright," by Herman A. Witkin; SCIENTIFIC AMERICAN, February, 1959; Offprint 410].

Merely informing an observer that a figure is tilted will often enable him to perceive the figure correctly. This may explain why some readers will not perceive certain of the rotated figures shown here as being strange or different. The converse situation, misinforming an observer about the figures, produces impressive results. If a subject is told that the top of a figure he is about to see is somewhere other than in the region uppermost in the environment, he is likely not to recognize the figure when it is presented with the orientation in which he first saw it. The figure is not disoriented and the observer incorrectly assigns the directions top, bottom and sides on the basis of instructions.

Since such knowledge about orientation will enable the observer to shift the directions he assigns to a figure, and since it is this assignment that affects the perception of shape, it is absolutely essential to employ naïve subjects in perception experiments involving orientation. That is, the subject must not realize that the experiment is concerned with figural orientation, so that he does not examine the figures with the intent of finding the regions that had been top, bottom, and sides in previous viewings of it. There are, however, some figures that seem to have intrinsic orientation in that regardless of how they are presented a certain region will be perceived as the top (see Figure 7.10). It is therefore difficult or impossible to adversely affect the recognition of such figures by disorienting them.

In the absence of other clues a subject will assign top-bottom coordinates according to his subjective or egocentric reference system. Consider a figure drawn on a circular sheet of paper that is lying on the ground. Neither gravity nor visual clues indicate where the top and bottom are. Nevertheless, an observer will assign a top to that region of the figure which is uppermost with respect to his egocentric coordinate reference system. The vertical axis of the figure is seen as being aligned with the long axis of

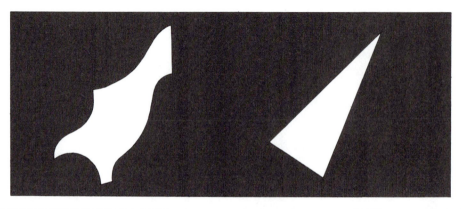

Figure 7.10 FIGURES WITH INTRINSIC ORIENTATION appear to have a natural vertical axis regardless of their physical orientation. A region at one end of the axis is perceived as top.

the observer's head and body. The upward direction corresponds to the position of his head. We have been able to demonstrate that such assignment of direction has the same effect on the recognition that other bases of assigning direction do. A figure first seen in one orientation on the circular sheet will generally not be recognized if its egocentric orientation is altered.

Now we come to an observation that seems to be at variance with much of what I have described. When a person lies on his side in bed to read, he does not hold the book upright (in the environmental sense) but tilts it. If the book is not tilted, the retinal image is disoriented and reading is quite difficult. Similarly, if a reader views printed matter or photographs of faces that are environmentally upright with his head between his legs, they will be just as difficult to recognize as they are when they are upside down and the viewer's head is upright. The upright pictures, however, are still perceived as being upright even when the viewer's head is inverted. Conversely, if the pictures are upside down in the environment and are viewed with the head inverted between the legs, there is no difficulty in recognizing them. Yet the observer perceives the pictures as being inverted. Therefore in these cases it is the orientation of the retinal image and not the environmental assignment of direction that seems to be responsible for recognition or failure of recognition.

Experiments with ambiguous figures conducted by Robert Thouless, G. Kanizsa and G. Tampieri support the notion that retinal orientation plays a role in recognition of a figure (see Figure 7.11). Moreover, as George Steinfeld and I have demonstrated, the recognition of upright words and faces falls off in direct proportion to the degree of body tilt (see Figure 7.12). With such visual material recognition is an inverse function of the degree of disorientation of the retinal image. As we have seen, the relation between degree of disorientation and recognizability does not hold in cases where the assignment of direction has been altered. In such cases the greatest effect is not with a 180-degree change but with a 45- or 90-degree change.

The results of all these experiments have led me to conclude that there are two distinct factors involved in the perception of disoriented figures: an assignment-of-direction factor and a retinal factor. I believe that when we view a figure with our head tilted, we automatically compensate for the tilt in much the same way that we compensate for the size of distal objects. An object at a moderate distance from us does not appear small in spite of the fact that its retinal image is much smaller than it is when the object is close by. This effect usually is explained by saying that the information supplied by the retinal image is somehow corrected by allowing for the distance of the object from us. Similarly, when a vertical luminous line in a dark room is viewed by a

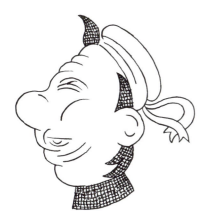 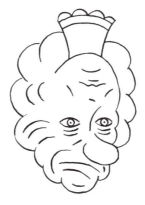 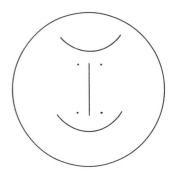

Figure 7.11 AMBIGUOUS FACES are perceived differently when their images on the retina of the observer are inverted. If you hold the illustration upright and view it from between your legs with your head inverted, the alternative faces will be perceived even though they are upside down in terms of the environment. The same effect occurs when the illustration is inverted and viewed from an upright position. Such tests provide evidence that figures such as faces are recognized on the basis of their upright retinal orientation.

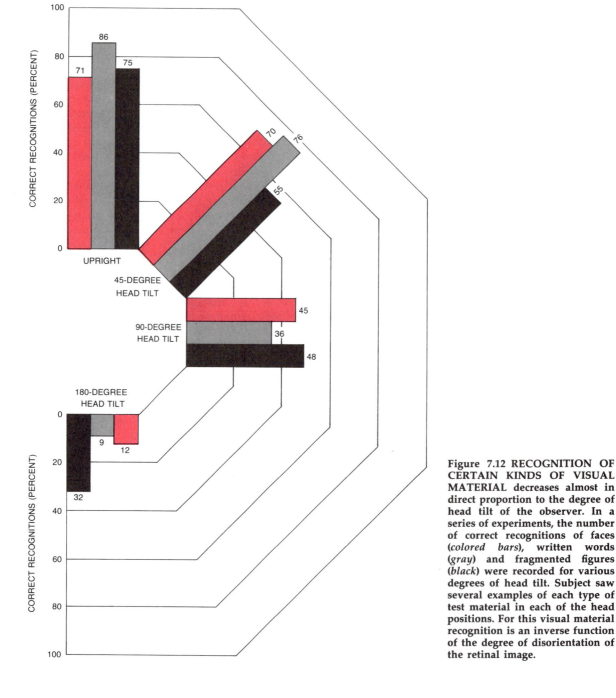

Figure 7.12 RECOGNITION OF CERTAIN KINDS OF VISUAL MATERIAL decreases almost in direct proportion to the degree of head tilt of the observer. In a series of experiments, the number of correct recognitions of faces (*colored bars*), written words (*gray*) and fragmented figures (*black*) were recorded for various degrees of head tilt. Subject saw several examples of each type of test material in each of the head positions. For this visual material recognition is an inverse function of the degree of disorientation of the retinal image.

tilted observer, it will still look vertical or almost vertical in spite of the fact that the retinal image in the observer's eye is tilted. Thus the tilt of the body must be taken into account by the perceptual system. The tilted retinal image is then corrected, with the result that the line is perceived as being vertical. Just as the correction for size at a distance is called size constancy, so can correction for the vertical be called orientation constancy.

When we view an upright figure with our head

tilted, before we have made any correction, we begin with the information provided by an image of the figure in a particular retinal orientation. The first thing that must happen is that the perceptual system processes the retinal image on the basis of an egocentrically assigned top, bottom and sides, perhaps because of a primitive sense of orientation derived from retinal orientation. For example, when we view an upright square with our head tilted, which yields a diamondlike retinal image, we may perceive a diamond for a fleeting moment before the correction goes into operation. Head orientation is then automatically taken into account to correct the perception. Thus the true top of the figure is seen to be one of the sides of the square rather than a corner. The figure is then "described" correctly as one whose sides are horizontal and vertical in the environment, in short as a "square." This correction is made quickly and usually without effort. In order to describe a figure the viewer probably must visualize or imagine it in terms of its true top, bottom and sides rather than in terms of its retinal top, bottom and sides.

If the figure is relatively simple, the correction is not too difficult to achieve. If we view an upright letter with our head tilted, we recognize it easily; it is of interest, however, that there is still something strange about it. I believe the dual aspect of the perception of orientation is responsible for this strangeness. There is an uncorrected perception of the letter based on its retinal-egocentric orientation and a corrected perception of it based on its environmental orientation. The first perception produces an unfamiliar shape, which accounts for the strange appearance of the letter in spite of its subsequent recognition. In our experiments many of the figures we employed were structurally speaking

equivalent to letters, and in some cases we actually used letters from unfamiliar alphabets (see Figure 7.13).

With a more complex figure, such as an inverted word or an upright word viewed by an observer, the corrective mechanism may be entirely overtaxed. Each letter of the word must be corrected separately, and the corrective mechanism apparently cannot cope simultaneously with multiple components. It is true that if an observer is given enough time, an inverted word can be deciphered, but it will never look the same as it does when it is upright. While one letter is being corrected the others continue to be perceived in their uncorrected form. There is a further difficulty: letter order is crucial for word recognition, and inverting a word reverses the normal left-to-right order.

The recognition of inverted longhand writing is even more difficult (see Figure 7.14). When such writing is turned upside down, many of the inverted "units" strongly resemble normal upright longhand letters. Moreover, since the letters are connected, it is difficult to tell where one letter ends and another begins. Separating the letters of the inverted word makes recognition easier. Even so, it is all too easy to confuse a *u* and an *n*. This type of confusion is also encountered with certain printed letters, namely, *b* and *q*, *d* and *p* and *n* and *u*, although not as frequently. In other words, if a figure is recognized on the basis of its upright retinal-egocentric orientation, this may tend to stabilize the perception and block the correction process. The dominance of the retinally upright faces in Figure 7.1 probably is an effect of just this kind.

There may be a similar overtaxing of the corrective mechanism when we view an inverted face. It

Figure 7.13 SINGLE LETTER that is tilted can be easily identified once it is realized how it is oriented. A strangeness in its appearance, however, remains because the per- cept arising from the uncorrected retinal image continues to exist simultaneously with the corrected percept.

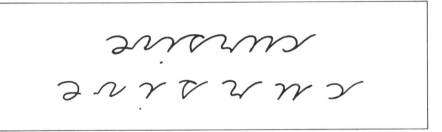

Figure 7.14 INVERTED LONGHAND WRITING is difficult to decipher because many inverted units resemble written upright letters. For example, an inverted *u* will look like an *n* and an inverted *c* like an *s*. Moreover, the connection between letters leads to uncertainty about where a letter begins and ends. Several inverted units can be grouped together and misperceived as an upright letter. Separating the inverted letters makes them easier to decipher.

may be that the face contains a number of features each of which must be properly perceived if the whole is to be recognized [see "The Recognition of Faces," by Leon D. Harmon; SCIENTIFIC AMERICAN, November, 1973; Offprint 555]. While attention is focused on correcting one feature, say the mouth, other features remain uncorrected and continue to be perceived on the basis of the image they form on the retina. Of course, the relation of features is also important in the recognition of a face, but here too there are a great number of such relations and the corrective mechanism may again be overtaxed. (See Figure 7.15).

Charles C. Bebber, Douglas Blewett and I conducted an experiment to test the hypothesis that it is the presence of multiple components that creates the difficulty of correcting figures. Subjects were briefly shown a quadrilateral figure and asked to study it. They viewed the target figure with their head upright. Then they were shown a series of test cards each of which had four quadrilateral figures. The test cards were viewed for one second, and the subjects were required to indicate if the target figure was on the card.

The subjects understood that they were to respond affirmatively only when they saw a figure that was identical with the target figure both in shape and in orientation. (Some of the test figures were similar to the target figure but were rotated by 180 degrees.) Half of the test cards were seen with

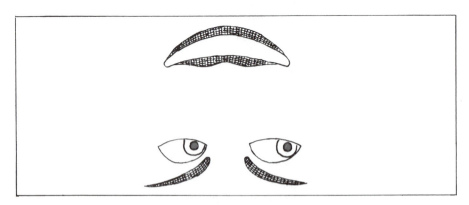

Figure 7.15 INVERTED FACIAL FEATURES are difficult to interpret because while attention is focused on correcting one feature, other features remain uncorrected. For example, one might succeed in correcting the eyes shown here so that they are perceived as gazing downward and leftward, but at that very moment the mouth is uncorrected and expresses sorrow rather than pleasure. Conversely, one might correct the mouth and misperceive the eyes.

the subject's head upright and half with the subject's head inverted. It was assumed that the subject would not be able to correct all four test figures in the brief time that was allowed him while he was viewing them with his head down. He had to perceive just as many units in the same brief time while he was viewing them with his head upright, but he did not have to correct any of the units. We expected that target figures would often not be recognized and that incorrect figures would be mistakenly identified as the target when the subjects viewed the test cards with their head inverted (see Figure 7.16).

The results bore out our prediction. When multiple components have to be corrected, retinal disorientation has an adverse effect on recognition. The observer responded to twice as many test cards correctly when he was upright than he did when he was inverted.

As I have noted, when we look at figures that are difficult to recognize when they are retinally disoriented, the difficulty increases as the degree of disorientation increases. Why this happens may also be related to the nature of the correction process. I suggested that the observer must suppress the retinally (egocentrically) upright percept and substitute a corrected percept. To do this, however, he must visualize or imagine how the figure would look if it were rotated until it was upright with respect to himself or, what amounts to the same thing, how it would look if he rotated himself into alignment with the figure. The process of mental rotation requires visualizing the entire sequence of angular change, and therefore the greater the angular change, the greater the difficulty.

As every parent knows, children between the ages of two and five seem to be quite indifferent to how a picture is oriented. They often hold a book upside down and seem not at all disturbed by it. On the basis of such observations and the results of some early experiments, many psychologists concluded that the orientation of a figure did not enter into its recognition by young children. More recent laboratory experiments, however, do not confirm the fact that children recognize figures equally well in any orientation. They have as much difficulty as, or more difficulty than, adults in recognizing previously seen figures when the figure is shown in a new orientation. Why then do young children often spontaneously look at pictures upside down in everyday situations? Perhaps they have not yet learned to pay attention to orientation, and do not realize that their recognition would improve if they did so. When children learn to read after the age of six, they are forced to pay attention to orientation because certain letters differ only in their orientation.

In summary, the central fact we have learned about orientation is that the perceived shape of a figure is not simply a function of its internal geometry. The perceived shape is also very much a function of the up, down and side directions we assign

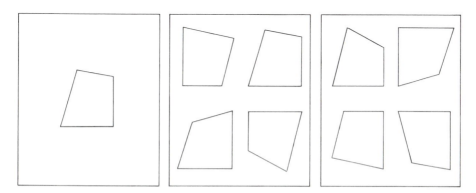

Figure 7.16 MULTIPLE ITEMS were found to have an adverse effect on recognition of even simple figures. Subjects sitting upright viewed the target (*left*). Then they were briefly shown test cards; some contained the target figure (*middle*) and some did not (*right*). The subjects were to indicate when they saw a figure that was identical with the target figure. Half of the test cards were viewed with the head upright and half with the head inverted. Recognition was poor when inverted subjects viewed the test cards. In other experiments with a single test figure head inversion did not significantly affect recognition.

to the figure. If there is a change in the assigned directions, the figure will take on a different perceptual shape. I have speculated that the change in perceived shape is based on a new "description" of the figure by the perceptual system. The directions assigned are based on information of various kinds about where the top, bottom and sides of a figure are and usually do not depend on the retinal orientation of the image of the figure. When the image is not retinally upright, a process of correction is necessary in order to arrive at the correct description, and this correction is difficult or impossible to achieve in the case of visual material that has multiple components.

All of this implies that form perception in general is based to a much greater extent on cognitive processes than any current theory maintains. A prevailing view among psychologists and sensory physiologists is that form perception can be reduced to the perception of contours and that contour perception in turn can be reduced to abrupt differences in light intensity that cause certain neural units in the retina and brain to fire. If this is true, then perceiving form results from the specific concatenation of perceived contours. Although the work I have described does not deny the possible importance of contour detection as a basis of form perception, it does suggest that such an explanation is far from sufficient, and that the perception of form depends on certain mental processes such as description and correction. These processes in turn are necessary to account for the further step of recognition of a figure. A physically unchanged retinal image often will not lead to recognition if there has been a shift in the assigned directions. Conversely, if there has been no shift in the assigned directions, even a very different retinal image will still allow recognition.

Perceiving Shape from Shading

Shading produces a compelling perception of three-dimensional shape. One way the brain simplifies the task of interpreting shading is by assuming a single light source.

· · ·

Vilayanur S. Ramachandran
August, 1988

Our visual experience of the world is based on two-dimensional images: flat patterns of varying light intensity and color falling on a single plane of cells in the retina. Yet we come to perceive solidity and depth. We can do this because a number of cues about depth are available in the retinal image: shading, perspective, occlusion of one object by another and stereoscopic disparity. In some mysterious way the brain is able to exploit these cues to recover the three-dimensional shapes of objects.

Of the many mechanisms employed by the visual system to recover the third dimension, the ability to exploit shading is probably the most primitive. One reason for believing this is that in the natural world many animals have evolved pale undersides, presumably to make themselves less visible to predators. "Countershading" compensates for the shading effects caused by the sun shining from above and has at least two benefits: it reduces the contrast with the background and it "flattens" the animal's perceived shape. The prevalence of countershading in a variety of species, including many fishes, suggests that shading may be a crucial source of information about three-dimensional shape.

Painters, of course, have long exploited lighting and shading to convey vivid illusions of depth. Psychologists, however, have not devoted much research to uncovering the mechanisms by which the eye and the brain actually take advantage of shading information. My colleagues and I therefore embarked on a set of experiments intended to reveal what some of the mechanisms might be.

We started out by creating a set of computer-generated displays of simple objects in which subtle variations in shading alone convey the impression of depth. We made sure the images were devoid of any complex objects and patterns, because our goal was to isolate the brain mechanisms that process shading information from higher-level mechanisms that may also contribute to depth perception in real-life visual processing.

Our experiments were based on circular, shaded shapes that create a compelling sensation of depth (see Figure 8.2a). The shapes either pop outward like eggs or inward like the cavities of an egg carton. The shapes are ambiguous because the brain does not know from which direction the light is shining. With some effort you can mentally shift the light source to invert the depth of the objects.

Intriguingly, when you mentally reverse the depth of one object, all the other objects in the display reverse simultaneously. This raises an inter-

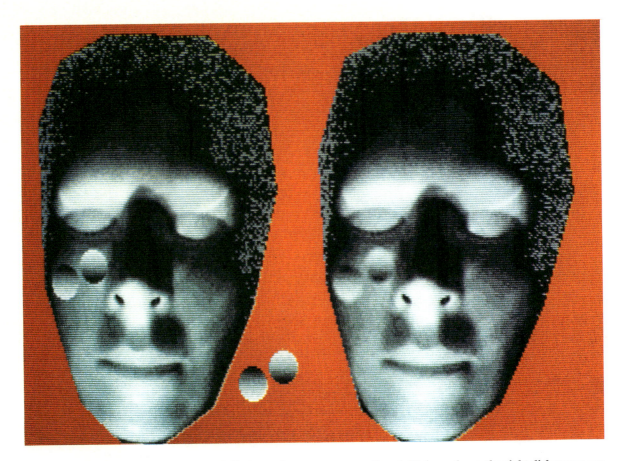

Figure 8.1 HOLLOW-MASK INTERIORS lit from above produce an eerie impression of protruding faces lit from below. In interpreting shaded images the brain usually assumes light shining from above, but here it rejects the assumption in order to interpret the images as normal, convex objects. Notice the two disks near the chin still appear as though lit from above: the right disk seems convex and the left one concave. When the disks are pasted on the cheek (*left*), their depth becomes ambiguous. When blended into the cheek (*right*), the disks are seen as being illuminated from below, like the rest of the face.

esting question: Is the propensity for seeing all objects in the display as being simultaneously convex (or concave) based on a tendency to see all of them as having the same depth or is it based on the tacit assumption that there is only one light source? To find out, we created a display in which objects in one row are mirror images of objects in the other row (see Figure 8.2*b*). In this display, when subjects see one row of objects as convex, they always perceive the other as concave.

We drew two conclusions from this simple experiment. First, the derivation of shape from shading cannot be a strictly local operation; it must be a global process involving either the entire visual field or a large portion of it. Second, the visual system seems indeed to assume that only one light source illuminates the entire image. This may be because our brains evolved in a solar system that has only one sun.

Another manifestation of this rule is seen in a complex shape suggesting a white tube lit from the side (see Figure 8.2*c*). The shape nearly always appears convex, perhaps because of subtle cues such as the occlusion of one part of the tube by another, or because of a general tendency to see such shapes as convex. Interestingly, the depth of the two disks

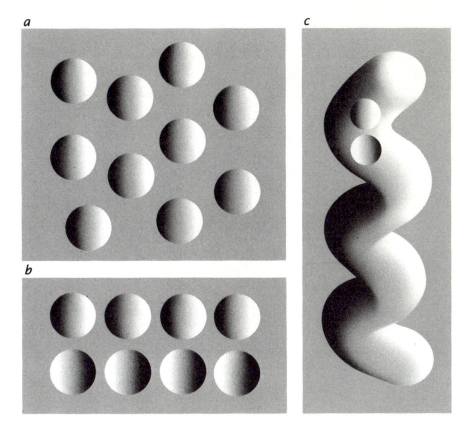

Figure 8.2 SPHERES OR CAVITIES? You can reverse the depth of the objects (*a*) by mentally shifting the light source from left to right. In a second array (*b*) each row by itself is ambiguous, but once you see one row as convex, the other row will always appear concave. It is almost impossible to see both as simultaneously convex or con-cave. The convoluted form (*c*) suggests a white tube lit from the right. The two disks seems to conform to the lighting scheme; the top disk is seen as a bump, the bottom one as a cavity. (The convoluted form experiment was done in collaboration with Dorothy Kleffner and Steven J. Cobb.)

superposed on the tube is no longer ambiguous; one is clearly a bump and the other a cavity. Apparently certain features of an object can inform the brain about the direction of illumination, and the depth of other parts of the object are then made to conform to the light source.

The visual system not only assumes a single light source but also tends to assume, naturally enough, that the light comes from above. We vividly demonstrate this effect with a display in which one group of shaded circles is simply the upside-down version of another group (see Figure 8.3) Subjects always perceive group *a* as consisting of spheres and group *b* as consisting of cavities. If you turn the page upside down, you will find a striking reversal of

depth: the objects in group *b* now appear convex and those in group *a* appear concave. (You can amuse yourself by cutting out the illustration and mounting it on a turntable. How fast can you spin the turntable before you stop seeing the reversals?)

These observations suggest that the brain assumes the sun shines from above. But how does the brain know "above" from "below"? Is it the object's orientation in relation to the retina that matters, or is it its orientation with respect to the external world? To appreciate this point try the following experiment. Lie on a couch and let your head hang over the edge so that you are looking at the world upside down. Now ask a friend to stand behind your head and hold Figure 8.3 upright. The objects in group *a*

a

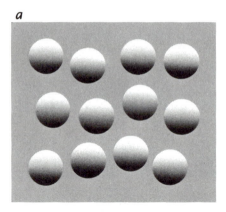

b

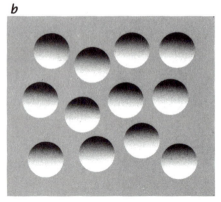

Figure 8.3 BRAIN ASSUMES light comes from above. The objects in group *a* therefore appear convex, whereas those in group *b* appear concave. If you turn the page upside down, the objects will reverse in depth. By turning your head upside down and looking at the page, you can prove it is the orientation of the pattern on the retina that matters.

will look concave and those in group *b* convex; that is, you get the same effect as you did when you rotated the page. Thus it is the orientation of the object on the retina that matters. Your objective knowledge of up and down does not affect your perception of depth.

Shading by itself generates only a weak impression of three-dimensional shape. To convey a convincing impression of depth the shaded surface must also be enclosed by an outline. Indeed, in many of our displays the luminance variation only roughly approximates the smooth, cosine variation of true shading, and yet the mere presence of a circular outline around the shaded region can generate a compelling illusion of a spherical surface. This raises a new question: What is the exact role of the outline in determining the perception of shape from shading?

To answer the question, we designed a pair of objects that have the same shading but different outlines (see Figure 8.4). Both images have the same luminance gradient: a photocell dragged across each image would register identical variations in the distribution of luminance. Yet the images are strikingly different. The upper image suggests three cylinders lying side by side, whereas the lower image conveys the unmistakable impression of a sheet of corrugated metal. The perceptions seem to depend completely on the contours of the top and bottom edges of the surfaces.

We conclude from these demonstrations that when shading cues are ambiguous, information from borders helps to resolve ambiguity throughout the image. Interestingly, the perceived location of the light source also shifts to conform to the perceived surface. In the upper image in Figure 8.4 the light seems to originate perpendicular to the page whereas in the lower image the illumination is from the far left or the far right. It is remarkable that changing an object's boundaries can produce such striking changes in perception.

Our next demonstration shows that even illusory contours will work. A typical example consists of four dark gray disks with a "bite" taken out of each one (see Figure 8.5). When the disks are in proper alignment, one has the impression of a large pale disk at the center partially occluding the gray disks. Indeed, faint lines seem to connect the concave edges of the gray disks, although such lines do not exist physically.

What happens if we replace the background of this display with one in which the luminance varies from top to bottom? (See Figure 8.5*b*.) The new display looks flat at first, but on prolonged viewing the region inside the illusory disk starts to bulge out toward the observer and may even detach itself from the background to take on the appearance of a floating sphere. Oddly enough, an illusory contour seems to work even better than a real outline (see Figure 8.5*c*.) The reason is not entirely clear but the result suggests that the brain regards partial occlusion as stronger evidence for the existence of an object than the presence of a mere outline. After all,

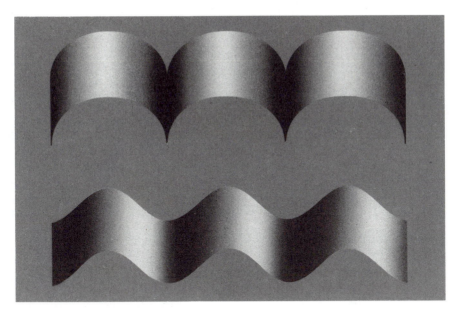

Figure 8.4 BOUNDARIES influence the interpretation of shaded surfaces. Both images have the same shading variation but the top image suggests three cylinders lit vertically to the page and the bottom one a corrugated metal sheet lit from far left (or far right).

the outline might equally well depict a loop of thin wire or a transparent soap bubble.

This observation, like the preceding one, demonstrates a direct and powerful interaction between edges, whether real or illusory, and the derivation of shape from shading. If the visual system were making detailed measurements of shading alone to recover surface orientation (as is implied in some artificial-intelligence models of vision), one would not see a sphere in the image, because the shading does not change at all across the illusory border. Yet the visual system perceives a sphere because the shading and the illusory outline mutually reinforce that interpretation.

Another way the visual system delineates objects is by changes in surface reflectance, or the proportion of light reflected by surfaces. A photocell moving across an object's border will usually register an abrupt shift in luminance. What would happen if the outline were defined by a change of color rather than a change of luminance? We took a typical shaded "sphere" and replaced the homogeneous gray background with a colored background in which the luminance gradient matched that of the sphere (see Figure 8.5e). The result was dramatic: the illusion of depth dissolved and the sphere ap

peared flattened, even though its outline was distinctly visible because of the contrast in hue. We concluded that the shape-from-shading system cannot make use of edges defined by color differences. One reason may be that our primitive primate ancestors, which resembled tarsiers, were nocturnal and color-blind; in their twilight world they relied on luminance contrast alone to perceive depth.

These demonstrations imply that the brain recovers information about the shape of objects by combining outlines and shading cues. What does the brain do with the shapes once it has recovered them? An important capacity of perception is the ability to segregate figure from ground. Even in a cluttered scene the visual system can easily decide which features in the image belong together to form objects. In a high-contrast photograph one can see a Dalmation dog against a dappled background (see Figure 8.6a). Similarly, one can mentally "lift out" a group of lines that have a particular orientation from a field of lines with a different orientation (see Figure 8.6b). On the other hand, it is impossible to segregate a group of mirror-reversed letters from unreversed ones (see Figure 8.6c).

The laws of perceptual grouping uncovered by

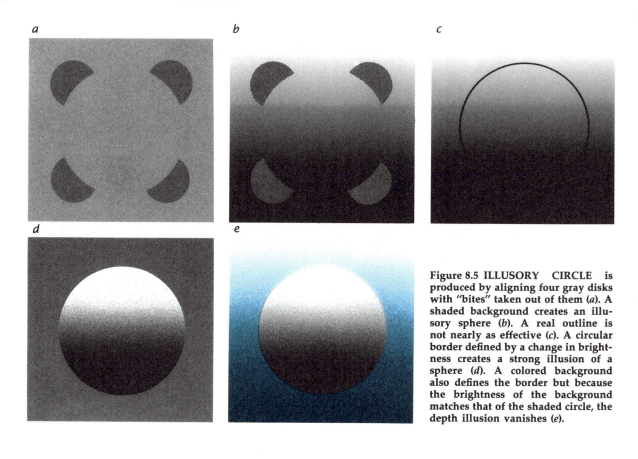

Figure 8.5 ILLUSORY CIRCLE is produced by aligning four gray disks with "bites" taken out of them (a). A shaded background creates an illusory sphere (b). A real outline is not nearly as effective (c). A circular border defined by a change in brightness creates a strong illusion of a sphere (d). A colored background also defines the border but because the brightness of the background matches that of the shaded circle, the depth illusion vanishes (e).

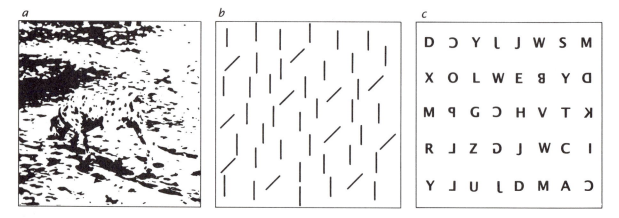

Figure 8.6 PERCEPTUAL GROUPING of elementary features enables one to segregate the shape of a Dalmatian dog from a speckled ground in a high-contrast photograph (a). Slanted lines can be grouped and envisioned as occupying a separate plane from vertical lines (b). Mirror-reversed letters, however, cannot be visually grouped and segregated from normal letters (c).

the Gestalt psychologists were later studied system-atically by Anne M. Treisman of the University of California at Berkeley, Bela Julesz then at AT&T Bell Laboratories and Jacob Beck of the University of Oregon. These investigators discovered several im-portant principles. First, they found than an impor-tant early stage of visual perception involves ex-tracting certain elementary features, which Julesz calls textons. Examples include oriented edges, color and direction of movement. Once the visual system has extracted the elementary features, similar fea-tures are grouped together to form objects. Indeed, Beck suggests that only elementary features, by def-inition, can be grouped in this way. Presumably, then, alphabetic characters are not elementary fea-tures as far as the visual system is concerned.

What about three-dimensional objects, though? Our next several demonstrations show that even shapes defined exclusively by shading can serve as elementary features of visual perception. In an array of cavities interspersed with convex shapes, for ex-ample, the convex shapes can mentally be grouped together to form a separate depth plane that is clearly segregated from the concave shapes in the background (see Figure 8.7a).

When one views this display, it appears as though the visual system passes through several stages of processing. In the earliest stage the system performs computations of redefining the three-dimensional shapes, taking several seconds. Once the convex shapes have emerged, one has the distinct impres-sion of being able to "hold on" to them indefinitely in order to group them with similar items in the display. Finally, after the objects are grouped, they are clearly segregated from irrelevant items in the background. The extraction and grouping of tex-tons, then, although usually described as a one-step operation, may in fact involve several distinct per-ceptual capacities that act together to delineate fig-ure from ground.

We wondered whether the perceptual grouping observed in that display might be the result of some other, more elementary feature than the three-di-mensional shape. For example, because the convex shapes differ from the concave ones in the polarity of their bright-to-dark luminance, one might sup-pose the grouping is achieved by latching on to luminance polarity. To rule out this possibility, we created a display of objects that have the same lumi-nance polarities as those in the preceding display but that do not carry any depth information (see Figure 8.7b). It is virtually impossible to achieve

perceptual grouping in this display. Even after you have spotted all the targets individually, you will not be able to segregate them from the rest of the objects. Clearly the grouping observed in the pre-ceding display must be based on three-dimensional shape rather than on luminance polarity.

I have pointed out that the illusion of depth is much more powerful when the illumination is from above than when it seems to come from the side. Similarly, lighting from above greatly enhances one's ability to group and segregate images. You can verify this by simply rotating group a in Figure 8.7 by 90 degrees: the impression of depth will dimin-ish and there will be a considerable reduction in perceptual segregation. This further supports the idea that perceptual grouping must be based on three-dimensional shape. Moreover, these group-ings can themselves represent higher-level shapes, such as a triangle (see Figure 8.7c). It might be interesting to employ stimuli of this kind to find out whether infants and brain-damaged patients can perceive shape from shading; for example, would an infant respond to spheres arranged to suggest a face?

Another remarkable capacity of visual percep-tion is the ability to detect symmetry. This abil-ity extends to fairly complicated shapes, such as plants, faces and Rorschach inkblots. How does the visual system detect symmetry? Does it match all the individual features on one side with those on the other side to determine whether an object is symmetrical? Or does it group features into more meaningful shapes and then look for symmetry in those shapes? Our next demonstration is an attempt to answer these questions.

We compared two arrays of shaded circles (see Figure 8.8). Subjects usually perceived the left-hand array as spheres and cavities arranged symmetric-ally about a horizontal axis. Yet a point-by-point examination reveals that the bottom half of the array is not a mirror image of the top half. In fact, it is the array on the right that is truly symmetri-cal. These results imply that the perception of sym-metry is based on three-dimensional shape rather than on the simple distribution of bright and dark areas in the image. You can verify this by rotating the illustration 90 degrees to eliminate the strong impression of depth. You will now see that the right-hand array is more symmetrical than the left-hand one.

Our observations suggest that shading informa-

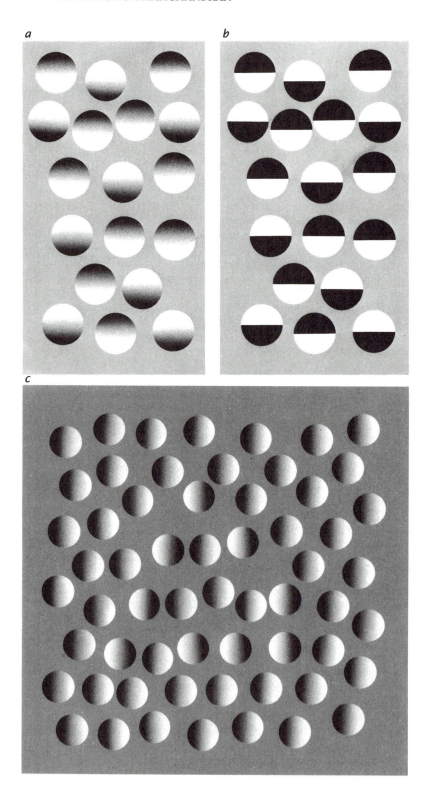

Figure 8.7 VISUAL SYSTEM can pick out convex shapes from concave ones and group them together (*a*). In an array that conveys the same luminance polarities as the preceding one but no depth information (*b*) it is impossible to visually segregate objects. In an array lit from the side (*c*), perceptual grouping becomes easier when you rotate the picture by 90 degrees. The convex objects stand out and form a triangle. Shading can define such complex shapes for further visual processing. A similar idea has been proposed by Alex Pentland of the Massachusetts Institute of Technology.

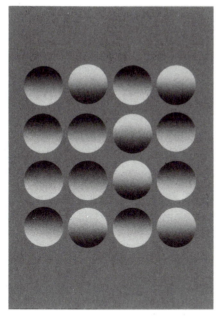 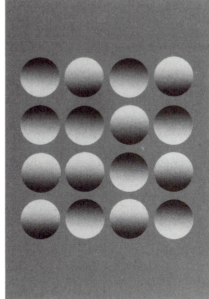

Figure 8.8 SYMMETRY PERCEPTION occurs after the brain extracts shape from shading. In the left-hand array, spheres and cavities seem arranged symmetrically about a horizontal axis. But in two dimensions it is the right-hand array that is truly symmetrical.

tion is extracted fairly early in visual processing. Indeed, there may even be neural channels specifically committed to the purpose. Recently Terrence J. Sejnowski and Sidney R. Lekhy of Johns Hopkins University raised the possibility that such cells may exist, based on work with a computer simulation. They began with a "neural network" consisting of three layers of cells: an input layer, a hidden layer and an output layer. Input-layer cells were modeled on the circular, "center surround" receptive fields of cells in a cat's eye. A learning algorithm adjusted the strength of signals passing from cells in one layer to the next, and after 40,000 trials the network could correctly associate shaded shapes with their three-dimensional axes of curvature.

What happened next came as a surprise: the investigators examined the responses of the cells in the hidden layer and found that they responded to bars of various lengths, widths and orientations, bearing an uncanny resemblance to edge-detector cells found in the visual cortex of cats and monkeys. Intriguing as this computer simulation is, its biological relevance is still not clear because the investigators deliberately excluded outlines and other cues known to play a crucial role in human vision. It remains to be seen whether the resemblance between the hidden units and the cortical edge detectors is merely a coincidence or whether edge-detector cells actually serve to extract three-dimensional shapes from shading.

I have so far considered stationary images, but what about moving objects? In nature it is a reasonably safe bet that anything that moves is either prey or predator. Consequently the visual system appears to have evolved a wide variety of mechanisms for detecting movement. Evidence suggests that the ability to see movement is mediated by specialized groups of brain cells. Can the brain mechanism enabling us to perceive motion also take advantage of information provided by shading? In order to find out we decided to exploit a well-known illusion called apparent motion (see Chapter 9, "The Perception of Apparent Motion," by Vilayanur S. Ramachandran and Stuart M. Anstis).

A simple example of apparent motion is produced by flashing two spatially separated spots of light in rapid alternation. Instead of seeing two lights flashing on and off one usually sees a single light jumping back and forth. To investigate the role of shading cues in human motion perception we created a display that alternated rapidly between one frame showing a shaded convex object above a concave one and a second frame in which the objects are reversed. Eleven naive subjects reported seeing a sphere jumping up and down between two holes in the background.

The result suggests that the brain must first compute three-dimensional shape before it can perceive apparent motion. Indeed, subjects often take tens of seconds to develop a depth impression, during which time they see no apparent motion. It therefore seems unlikely that the apparent motion could be based on some other, more primitive feature of the image. To demonstrate the point more directly we rotated the entire display by 90 degrees. This reduced the impression of depth considerably and led to an almost complete loss of the apparent-motion effect.

The visual system, then, appears to extract a three-dimensional object from shading cues and to perceive movement based on the three-dimensional image, rather than using the "primitive" two-dimensional image directly. Certain cells in the visual cortex of the monkey respond to the apparent motion of simple stimuli such as the flashing spots of light described above. It might be interesting to see whether these cells would respond to motion based on objects whose shape is perceived from shading.

Clearly, visual perception relies on a constellation of biological processes to arrive at a three-dimensional representation of the world. In order to create this representation the visual system appears to make a variety of simplifying assumptions, such as the rule that there is only one light source. What happens when the visual system tries to construct a coherent scene out of many disparate fragments? Patrick Cavanagh, Diane Rogers-Ramachandran and I recently did a study to try to answer the question.

We created simple arrays of randomly placed chevrons, each of which can be viewed as two adjoining faces of a cube. Array *a* (Figure 8.9) can be perceived as parallel cubes all pointing in the same direction and illuminated by a single light source; the black parallelograms are seen as the shadowed face of the cubes. But equally often the array is perceived as a set of white "gravestones" casting black shadows. By mentally shifting the direction of the light source you can switch from seeing cubes to seeing gravestones. Note that when you see any one

figure in the array as a cube you see all others as cubes too. It is impossible, in fact, to simultaneously perceive some figures as cubes and the others as gravestones, because such a perception would violate the single-light-source rule. Interestingly, when the shapes are perceived as cubes, there is a tendency to fill in the missing faces—that is, to perceive illusory surfaces. The illusory surfaces vanish when the shapes are seen as gravestones.

Next we randomly inverted or reversed roughly half of the chevrons in various combinations. These new displays illustrate the subtle interplay of constraints and organizing rules that occurs when the brain tries to create meaningful shapes from isolated fragments. In array *b* (Figure 8.9), for instance, all the targets usually appear as parallel cubes even though this would be incompatible with a single light source. Apparently when the single-light-source rule cannot be satisfied, it is replaced by a "pointing" rule (or by a rule stating that shapes with similar orientations are in fact parallel surfaces). To avoid conflict the brain simply assumes that the cubes have faces of differing color.

In array *c* (Figure 8.9) you will see a mixture of gravestones and cubes because this allows the system to satisfy the single-light-source rule. It is actually impossible to see the display as consisting entirely of cubes or of gravestones, because such a perception would not be compatible with either the pointing rule or the light-source rule. You will also find yourself unifying all the items in the array into a single coherent surface so that it suggests a sculptured metal surface with randomly placed "steps" carved out of it. Whereas an ant crawling on the picture would see only chaotic fluctuations in brightness, the human eye surveys the entire image and knits parallel surfaces together to create spatial order and unity.

In array *d* (Figure 8.9) the figures are neither parallel nor able to satisfy the single-light-source constraint. Hence there is a tendency to see the display as a random collection of flat chevrons pointing in opposite directions. Even though an individual figure in the display can sometimes be seen as a cube or a gravestone, it is difficult to unify all of them into a coherent three-dimensional interpretation.

In the real world, visual imagery—that is, high-level knowledge about what one is seeing—profoundly affects the perception of shape from shading. Indeed, the interaction between visual imagery and perception is one of the most elusive and

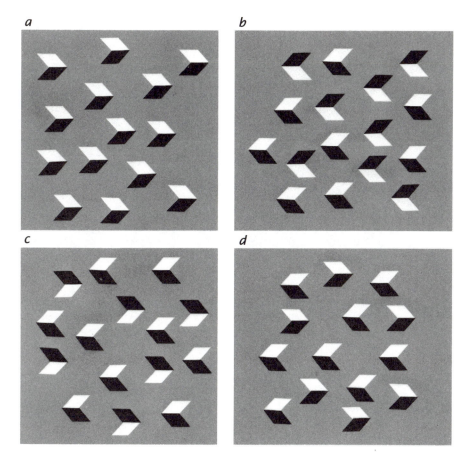

Figure 8.9 CHEVRONS in group *a* appear as illusory cubes or as "gravestones" casting shadows, all lit from the same angle. In group *b* a "pointing" rule seems to override the single-light-source rule and the image is seen as a set of cubes whose faces have different reflectances. Group *c* is always seen as a mixture of cubes and gravestones because this interpretation satisfies the single-light-source rule. Group *d* is ambiguous, and it is difficult to unify the figures into a coherent interpretation.

enigmatic topics in psychology. To illustrate this point, we created an array of shaded circles that on casual inspection appear to form alternating rows of spheres and cavities (see Figure 8.10). The display is susceptible to a radically different interpretation, however: it can be seen as a gray sheet with 16 holes cut out, behind which are two blurred, dark stripes. This perceptual switch causes the shaded circles to lose their spherical shape completely.

The tendency to see stripes rather than spheres and cavities can be enhanced by stereoscopic cues. You can see spheres in Figure 8.10*b*, but if you were to "fuse" them binocularly through a stereoscopic viewer, you would see a frame with a circular window standing out clearly from a shaded background. Indeed, it becomes virtually impossible to see the circular shape as a sphere instead of a hole. This implies that the extraction of shape from shading is strongly affected by stereoscopic processing.

The interpretation of shape from shading also interacts strongly with the visual system's knowledge of objects, as is strikingly demonstrated by the opening figure for this chapter (see Figure 8.1). In these photographs the hollow insides of face masks are illuminated from above; one would therefore expect them to look hollowed out. But the visual

a   *b*

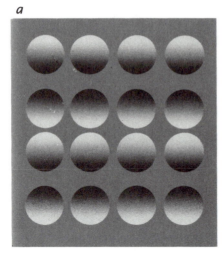
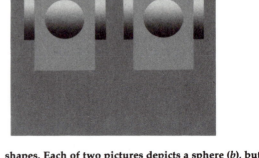

Figure 8.10 VISUAL IMAGERY, or higher-level informa-tion about objects, profoundly influences the perception of shape from shading. Rows of spheres and cavities (*a*) can also be seen as two blurred stripes visible through 16 holes cut in an opaque sheet. One can no longer see the spherical shapes. Each of two pictures depicts a sphere (*b*), but when they are "fused" in a stereoscopic viewer, the spheres van-ish and one sees a circular window cut in a rectangular sheet floating in front of a shaded plane.

system strongly rejects the possibility of hollow shapes and interprets the images as normal faces lit from below. Thus the visual system overrides the assumption of lighting from above in order to be able to interpret the shapes as normal faces.

Now notice the two small, shaded disks between the chins of the two faces. Even though the light on the faces is assumed to come from below, the disk on the right generally is seen as convex and the one on the left as concave—as though they were both illuminated from above. Perhaps the brain treats these objects as being quite distinct from the faces and therefore, in interpreting their shading, adheres to the more "primitive" rule that they are illumi-nated from above. When the disks are pasted onto the cheek of one of the faces, however, the depth becomes ambiguous: the right-hand disk can appear concave and the left-hand one convex. Finally, when the outlines of the disks are blended into the cheek, they are always seen as being illuminated from below, like the rest of the face. Consequently

the disk at the right suggests a dimple and the one at the left looks like a bump or a tumor.

Our research has revealed a variety of rules that are applied early in the visual processing of shape from shading. We have shown that it is possible to trace the flow of information from the very early stages of shape perception to the final stage, where the information interacts with high-level knowledge of light sources and of the nature of complex, three-dimensional objects. The neurological events me-diating the process in human beings are still myste-rious, but insights from psychology can help to elucidate what these events may be and how they are organized in the brain. New computational models can also offer plausible mechanisms and help to narrow the search. These developments are launching research on visual perception into a new domain, where it may someday be possible to dis-cover the cellular mechanisms in the brain that en-able us to perceive the world visually in three dimensions.

The Perception of Apparent Motion

When the motion of an intermittently seen object is ambiguous, the visual system resolves confusion by applying some tricks that reflect a built-in knowledge of properties of the physical world.

. . .

Vilayanur S. Ramachandran and Stuart M. Anstis
June, 1986

Producers of motion pictures, television programs and even neon signs have long banked on the fact that human beings have a quirk in their visual system. When it is confronted with a rapid series of still images, the mind can "fill in" the gaps between "frames" and imagine that it sees an object in continuous motion. For instance, a series of neon arrows lighted up in succession are perceived as being a single arrow moving through space. The illusion of continuous motion is called apparent motion to distinguish it from "real" motion, which is perceived when an object moves continuously across a viewer's visual field. When Sir Laurence Olivier appears to be fencing in a film, he is in apparent motion, whereas a person walking across the theater in front of the screen is in real motion. (See Figure 9.1.)

In the century or so since the motion picture was invented, filmmakers and television workers have learned to create many compelling illusions of motion, but their progress has been furthered mainly by rule-of-thumb empiricism. Psychological research is only now beginning to describe the mechanisms by which the visual system — the retina and the brain — perceives apparent motion.

The starting point of our own investigations was the premise, set forth by Bela Julesz working at AT&T Bell Laboratories and Oliver J. Braddick of the University of Cambridge, that to perceive an intermittently visible object as being in continuous motion the visual system must above all detect what is called correspondence. That is, it must determine which parts of successive images reflect a single object in motion. If each picture differs only slightly from the one before it, the visual system can perceive motion; if successive pictures differ greatly, the illusion of motion will be destroyed.

Our main question, then, was: How does the visual system go about detecting correspondence? One popular view holds that the brain does so by acting like a computer. When an image stimulates the retina, the eye transmits the image to the brain as an array of tiny points of varying brightness. The brain then compares each point to every point in succeeding frames. By means of complex computations the brain finally discerns the one set of matched points composing a single object that has changed its position — has moved. Attempts to build machines that "see" are generally based on this principle.

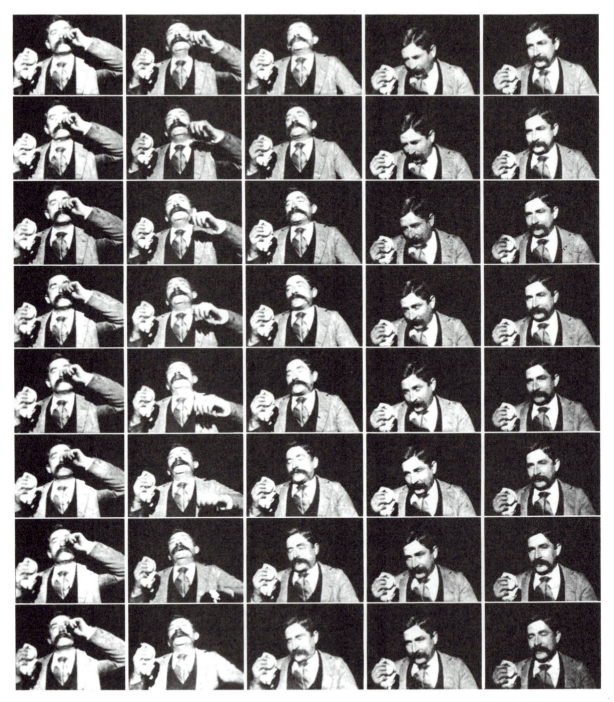

Figure 9.1 SUCCESSION OF FRAMES (*top to bottom, left to right*) capture a sneeze. They are from an early motion picture made in Thomas A. Edison's laboratory in about 1890. In order to perceive continuous motion when still images such as these are flashed, the visual system must above all detect correspondence; that is, it must identify elements in successive frames as being a single object in motion.

The scheme seems logical enough when a simple, unambiguous display is presented. For instance, if a small dot is shown in one frame and is followed by an identical dot placed slightly to the right, the visual system will readily identify the dot in the first frame as an object and find it again—displaced—in the second frame (see Figure 9.2a).

The scheme becomes problematical, however, when correspondence is to be detected in more intricate displays. For example, suppose two identical dots are shown in vertical alignment on a computer or television screen and are then replaced by congruent dots shifted to the right. In theory the visual system is now confronted with two possible correspondences: the dots in the first frame could be seen to jump horizontally along parallel paths to the right, or they could be seen to jump diagonally, in which case they would have to cross paths. In practice viewers always see the dots moving in parallel, never crossing (see Figure 9.2b).

In another display a computer-generated random-dot pattern forms the first image; then a square region is cut out of the middle and shifted horizontally to create the second image (see Figure 9.3). To the unaided eye the second image appears to be identical with the first and to have no separate central square. Now the images are superposed and then alternated rapidly so that the outer dots are in perfect register, or correlate, and so appear to be immobile. The middle region, where the dots are out of register, appears to move: a well-delineated

square is perceived to be oscillating from side to side.

To produce these two illusions by means of point-to-point matchings the brain would somehow need to invalidate hundreds of potential matches, deeming them to be false. While it is possible that the brain laboriously matches all the points and then subjects the matches to a series of elimination tests, our investigation suggests an entirely different approach to detecting correspondence: the visual system applies strategies that limit the number of matches the brain needs to consider and thereby avoids the need for complex point-to-point comparisons. (Computer-generated dot patterns were first introduced by Bela Julesz at AT&T Bell Laboratories and Donald M. MacKay of the University of Keele in England.)

We believe perception of apparent motion is controlled in the early stage of visual processing by what is in effect a bag of tricks, one the human visual system has acquired through natural selection during millions of years of evolution. Natural selection is inherently opportunistic. It is likely that the visual system adopted the proposed visual short cuts not for their mathematical elegance or aesthetic appeal, as some would suggest, but simply because they worked. (We call this idea the utilitarian theory of perception.) In the real world anything that moves is a potential predator or prey. Hence being able to quickly detect motion and determine

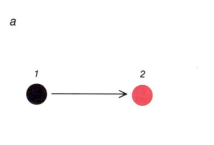

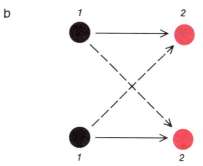

Figure 9.2 DOT DISPLAYS produce the illusion of motion. In a simple display (a) a spot of light (black) presented briefly is replaced by an identical spot displaced to the right (color). Numbers indicate the order of presentation. Rather then seeing two separate dots, the viewer perceives the first dot as moving horizontally (arrow). An ambiguous display (b) can be interpreted in two ways. Two vertically aligned dots (black) are flashed and then replaced by an identical pair displaced to the right (color). In theory the first dots can appear to move horizontally in parallel (solid arrows) or to move diagonally (broken arrows). In practice viewers always see the horizontal motion. The visual system detects correspondence by extracting salient features from images and limiting "legal" motions to those consistent with certain universal laws of matter and motion.

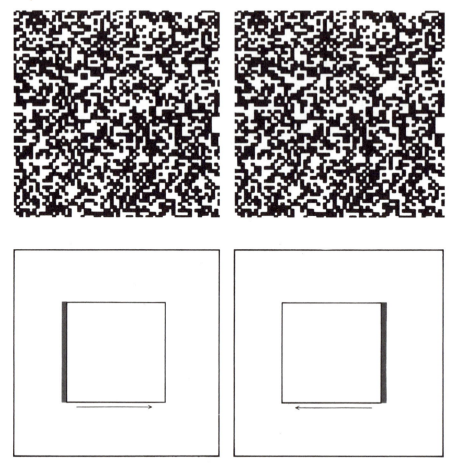

Figure 9.3 IMAGES COMPOSED OF RANDOM DOTS (*top*) produce apparent motion when they are superposed and then flashed alternately. The two computer-generated images are identical except that dots in a square central region of the second image (*right*) are shifted to the left with respect to their position in the first image (*left*), as is schematically shown (*bottom*). No central square is visible in either image alone, but when the images are alternated, a central square is seen oscillating horizontally against a stationary background.

what moved, and in what way, is crucial to survival. For example, the ability to see apparent motion between widely separated images may be particularly important when detecting the motion of animals that are seen intermittently, as when they move behind a screen of foliage or a tree trunk.

One trick of the visual system is to extract salient features, such as clusters of dots rather than individual dots, from a complex display and then search for just those features in successive images. This significantly reduces the number of potential matches and thus speeds the perceptual process;

after all, the probability that two chunks of a visual scene will be similar is much smaller than the probability that two points of brightness will be similar.

Among the features the visual system might attempt to extract from images are sharp outlines and edges or blotches of brightness and darkness; the latter are technically called areas of low spatial frequency. We have evaluated each of these and found that the visual system is likely to detect correspondence between regions of similar low spatial frequencies before it detects more detailed outlines or sharp edges. In other words, the visual system is likely to notice a dark blur moving in a forest long before it identifies the outline of an individual tree swaying in the breeze.

To demonstrate this principle we initially presented a white square on a black background for a tenth of a second and then replaced it with a congruent outline square to the left and a white circle to the right. (All the experiments described in this chapter presented images to viewers at speeds too fast for thinking; the objective was to eliminate the influence of high-order cognition and focus on the processes responsible for early perception.) Would the viewer see the white square move toward the outline square (which had the same sharp corners as the first square) or toward the circle (which had the same shading as the original square)? Subjects almost always saw the latter effect, providing evidence that the visual system tends to match areas of similar brightness in preference to matching sharp outlines (see Figure 9.4).

Texture is another feature that appears salient to the visual system. We and our colleagues at Stanley Medical College in Madras, India, presented to subjects two images of random-dot patterns; each image had an inner square with a visual texture different from that of the outer region (see Figure 9.5). The inner square of the second image was the same size and texture as the inner square of the first image, but it was rotated 90 degrees and was shifted horizontally.

We eliminated the possibility that correspondence could be detected on the basis of nontextural cues by ensuring that the dots in the two images would lack point-to-point correlation when the images were superposed and that the average brightness was the same in the inner and outer textures. We could therefore predict that if a shift of texture (such as between the inner and outer regions of the images) is a feature that enables the visual system to detect correspondence, viewers would see the inner square oscillating whenever the two images were alternated rapidly. If, on the other hand, texture is of no help in detecting correspondence, viewers would simply see visual "noise" and no coherent motion. Observers did see the oscillating square, indicating that texture is indeed an important cue for the detection of correspondence by a viewer.

Clearly the mechanism for perceiving apparent motion can accept various inputs for detecting correspondence. We have found a preference for seeing low spatial frequencies and textures; other investigators, such as Shimon Ullman of the Massachusetts Institute of Technology, have found that under certain circumstances line terminations and sharp edges also serve as cues. Perhaps the visual system perceives motion cues hierarchically, first scanning for coarse features before homing in on finer features, rather like an anatomist who first looks through a microscope set a low power before switching to higher magnification. One bit of evidence supporting this view is that subjects do indeed sometimes see the white square in the experiment cited above move toward the outline square, but only when the images are presented slowly and there is time to scrutinize the image.

In addition to extracting salient features a second trick of the visual system is to limit the matches it will consider to those yielding perceptions of mo-

Figure 9.4 FEATURES OF OBJECTS that might be extracted to detect correspondence are compared in this experiment. A solid square (*center*) is shown against a dark background and is then replaced with an outline square on the left and a solid circle on the right. The viewer who is confronted with these images usually sees the square move toward the circle rather than toward the outlined square, suggesting that regions of shadow or brightness (low spatial frequencies) are more likely to be detected initially than sharp edges or fine outlines.

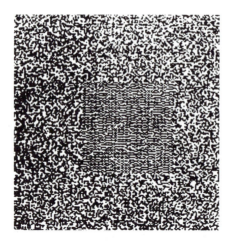

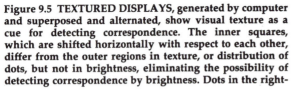

Figure 9.5 TEXTURED DISPLAYS, generated by computer and superposed and alternated, show visual texture as a cue for detecting correspondence. The inner squares, which are shifted horizontally with respect to each other, differ from the outer regions in texture, or distribution of dots, but not in brightness, eliminating the possibility of detecting correspondence by brightness. Dots in the right-hand image do not correlate with those in the other image, eliminating the possibility of detecting correspondence by point-to-point matching. Seeing an inner square oscillate horizontally when images are alternated can be explained only by the ability of the visual system to detect changes in texture.

tion that are sensible, or could occur in the real, three-dimensional world. In other words, as David Marr of MIT first suggested, the visual system assumes the physical world is not a chaotic and amorphous mess, and it capitalizes on the world's predictable physical properties. For instance, if the pairs of jumping dots described above were actually rocks, they would collide if they moved diagonally in the same depth plane and so would fail to reach opposite corners; the only logical perception of the dots' motion is therefore that the two dots in the first frame move in parallel to their positions in the second frame. Sure enough, when these dots are viewed through a stereoscope (a double-lens viewer) and seem to be in separate planes, observers do see them cross; in the real world, objects in different planes—such as airplanes at different altitudes—can indeed cross each other without colliding.

In order to examine the notion that the visual system assumes the world has order, we presented subjects with various motion displays that could be interpreted in more than one way and observed how subjects resolved the ambiguity. We found that one rule applied by the visual system is reminiscent of Isaac Newton's first law of motion, namely that objects in motion tend to continue their motion along a straight path. The visual system perceives linear motion in preference to perceiving abrupt changes of direction.

We demonstrated the power of this rule with an illusion that incorporated a "bistable (dual state) quartet": two dots briefly presented at diagonal corners of a square and then replaced by identical dots at the other two corners. A bistable quartet can be perceived in two ways, somewhat like the familiar Necker cube, which viewers see oscillating between two perspectives (see Figure 9.6). With approximately equal frequency observers of a bistable quartet see two dots oscillating horizontally or two dots oscillating vertically.

The bistable quartet was embedded in the center part of two horizontal rows of dots that appeared to be streaming in opposite directions (see Figure 9.7). Only one dot in each row was visible at a time. When the streaming dots reached the center of the screen, the bistable quartet became visible. At that point viewers could in theory see the dots continue in a horizontal path or could see them make a 90-degree turn followed by a second 90-degree turn, to produce two U-shaped trajectories. In practice observers invariably saw horizontal streaming, indicating that the tendency to see linear motion

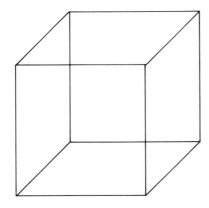

Figure 9.6 NECKER CUBE, named for the Swiss naturalist Louis A. Necker, can be seen to oscillate between two alternative perspectives.

overcame the ability to see the dots in the quartet move vertically. The U-shaped motion was seen only when the parallel rows were brought very close to each other; then Newton's law came in conflict with a competing tendency to see motion between the closest identical points. The proximity principle gains increasing power as objects are moved closer to each other.

A second rule that limits the possibilities for correspondence is that objects are assumed to be rigid; that is, all points on a moving object are assumed to move in synchrony. Image a leopard leaping from a branch of one tree to a branch of another. According to the rule of rigidity, the viewer who picks out any salient feature of the leopard, such as its basic shape (or even the splash of light shading, or low

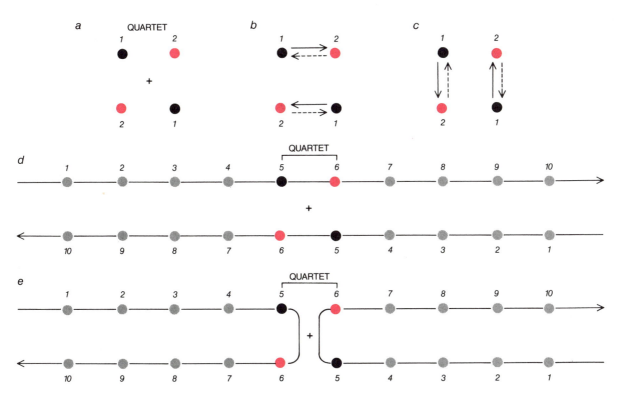

Figure 9.7 BISTABLE QUARTET, a square matrix of four dots (a), illustrates the visual system's tendency to see moving objects follow a straight path. Numbers indicate the order of presentation of dots on a screen; subjects are told to fix their gaze on the central cross. When dots at opposite corners (black) are flashed and then replaced by identical dots (color), viewers are equally likely to see the first dots move horizontally (b) or vertically (c). If two parallel rows of dots (d, e) are flashed in sequence (with two dots visible at a time), viewers can in theory see one of two trajectories (arrows) when the dots in the central, bistable quartet are flashed: horizontal "streaming" (d) or vertical "bouncing" along a U-shaped path (e). In practice, viewers invariably perceive streaming.

spatial frequency, of its coat), and finds the same feature in a second frame does not need to also compare every black spot on the animal. Without actually perceiving each leopard spot, the person assumes that all spots—indeed, all parts of the leopard—move in synchrony with the salient feature; correspondences suggesting that the leopard's spots can fly off in all directions are not even considered.

An experiment that demonstrated the rule of rigidity involved two uncorrelated random-dot pattern we alternated in a continuous cycle, exposing each picture for half a second (see Figure 9.8). Viewers saw random incoherent motion, much like "snow" on an untuned television set. Now we added a narrow strip of dots to the left of and abutting the edge of each image. The "grain" of the dots in the strips was the same as the grain in the images to which they were added, but the strip added to the second image was wider than the strip added to the first one, so that the left margins of the new images did not align. When the images were again alternated, the left margin appeared to shift from side to side. Strikingly, the entire display suddenly seemed to move in synchrony with the margin as a single solid sheet. We call this effect motion capture. Apparently unambiguous motion, such as

that seen at the left edge of the images, "captures" ambiguously moving fragments because the visual system tends to presume that all moving parts are fragments of a single object whose surface features move in synchrony.

A further experiment also demonstrated the phenomenon of captured motion, and particularly the ability of low spatial frequencies to effect such capture. We superposed blurred vertical bars of low-contrast lightness and darkness, called sine-wave gratings, on a pair of alternating and uncorrelated random-dot patterns (see Figure 9.9), so that ripple-like shadows seemed to move smoothly across the pattern. The moving shadows caused all the dots in the display to appear to move as a uniform sheet in step with the shadows.

The phenomenon of captured motion now enables us to explain how it is that an oscillating square can emerge when two images that individually do not appear to include a discrete central square are alternated (see Figure 9.3). Proponents of the computer analogy would contend that the illusion is a product of point-to-point matchings. It seems more plausible to suppose a viewer's visual system extracts a salient cluster of dots from the first display, finds it again in the second display and then assumes that all other "jumping" dots move in synchrony with the salient cluster. Such a short cut

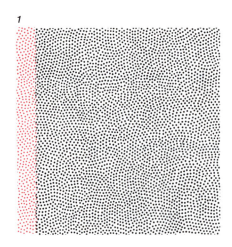

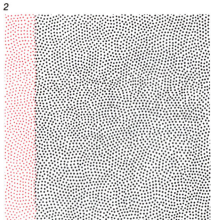

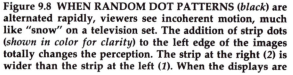

Figure 9.8 WHEN RANDOM DOT PATTERNS (black) are alternated rapidly, viewers see incoherent motion, much like "snow" on a television set. The addition of strip dots (shown in color for clarity) to the left edge of the images totally changes the perception. The strip at the right (2) is wider than the strip at the left (1). When the displays are alternated, viewers see the left margin oscillate horizontally and also see the entire display move in synchrony with the margin, a phenomenon known as motion capture. The visual system tends to see uniform motion and expects all parts of an object to move in synchrony with any salient part of the object.

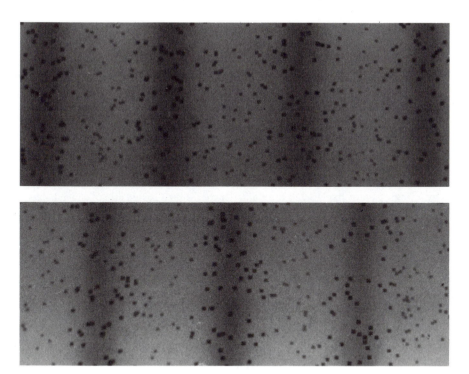

Figure 9.9 BLURRED LOW-CONTRAST BARS, components, of a so-called sine-wave grating, are shown superposed over random-dot displays that produce incoherent motion when they are themselves superposed and alternated in the absence of a grating. The addition of a grating that moves across the screen without ambiguity captures the motion of all the dots and causes them to move with the grating as a single sheet. This effect was studied by one of the authors (Ramachandran) together with Patrick Cavanagh of the University of Montreal.

would result in faster detection of correspondence than would comparing each point with every other point in successive images. A strategy of this kind would be particularly helpful in the real world, where additional salient features are usually found.

A third rule applied by the visual system, and something of a corollary to the other two, is that a moving object will progressively cover and uncover portions of a background. In other words, when matter, which is normally opaque, temporily occludes a background, the background still exists; it does not disappear.

Consider a display in which a triangle and a square below it are presented and then are replaced by another square adjacent to the triangle and directly to its right (see Figure 9.10a). One might expect to see the triangle and first square move toward the second square and fuse with it, or to see the first square alone move obliquely toward the second

square while the triangle just blinks on and off. In practice one sees something quite different: the triangle appears to move horizontally and to hide behind the obliquely moving square, which now appears to occlude a triangle that is not in fact being displayed. Clearly the brain turns to the real-world property of occlusion to explain the otherwise mysterious disappearance of the triangle. The continued existence of objects is accepted as a given by the visual system, even if the brain sometimes has to invent evidence to fulfill this expectation!

In a related experiment two dots of light in one frame were replaced in the second frame by a single dot, shifted to the right and parallel to the top dot. The images in the first frame seemed to converge at the image in the second frame (see Figure 9.10b). On the other hand, when a patch of tape or cardboard was added below the dot in the second frame, a new illusion was produced. Now observers saw the two dots move in parallel, with the bottom one

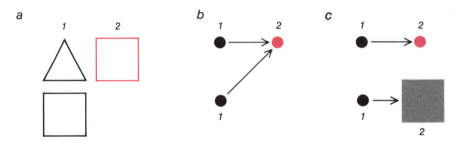

Figure 9.10 **TRIANGLE AND SQUARE** in one experiment (*a*) are presented simultaneously in one frame (*black*) and are then replaced by a single square displaced to the right (*color*). Numbers indicate the order of presentation. Subjects usually perceive the triangle as "hiding" behind a square that has moved to occlude it. In another experiment (*b*) two spots presented in the first frame (*black*) usually appear to move and fuse with the single spot displaced to the right in the second frame (*color*). If an opaque strip of paper is then pasted on the screen below the second dot (*c*), a new illusion of occlusion results: the lower spot appears to move horizontally and to hide behind the paper occluder.

hiding behind the patch, which was perceived to be an occluder (see Figure 9.10*c*). Once again the visual system tended to perceive the motion it was likely to find in the real world.

Yet another experiment demonstrated the power of the expectation that one object can occlude another. One of us (Ramachandran) showed viewers an image containing two clusters of four disks each (see Figure 9.11*a*). In one cluster a pie-shaped wedge was removed from each disk and in the other the disks were complete. We alternated this image with one in which the clusters were transposed. Subjects could in theory see four robotlike shapes, something like those in the game Pac-Mac, facing into the center with their "mouths" opening and closing; or viewers could imagine that the white space between the wedges formed a single oscillating square that first partially occluded and then

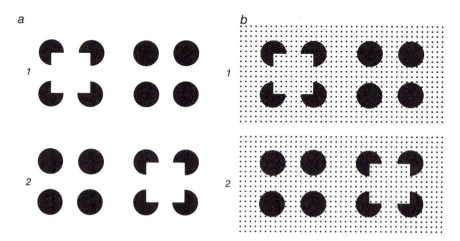

Figure 9.11 **DISK-SHAPED IMAGES** in computer displays produce illusions of occlusion and motion capture. In the images at the left (*a*) pie-shaped wedges are missing from four of eight black disks, first from the cluster of disks at the left (*1*) and then from the cluster at the right (*2*). When the two images are superposed and then alternated, viewers see a white square moving right and left, occluding and uncovering disks in the background. The images at the right (*b*) are identical with the first set but are presented against a background of stationary dots. When these images are alternated, viewers see the dots jump along with the oscillating square.

uncovered four disks. It turns out that the visual system interprets the images as an oscillating square, probably because in the three-dimensional world one is more likely to see a square shape occluding a background than see four identical robots opening and closing their mouths. The property of occlusion overrides any tendency to see movement between the closest similar objects. [The tendency of viewers to apply the rule of occlusion in resolving perceptual ambiguities also has been emphasized by Irvin Rock of the University of California at Berkeley.]

A slightly modified version of this stimulus illustrates the visual system's ability to combine strategies, in this case a predisposition to see both occlusion and rigidity in moving objects. When we superposed the alternating disk images on a background of stationary dots, viewers saw the illusory square oscillate as before, but now they also perceived a sheet of dots oscillating along with the square. The stationary dots were perceived to be a part of the square and therefore were "captured" by its apparent movement. Amazingly, the visual system sees all of this solely as the result of a change in just four tiny pie-shaped wedges (see Figure 9.11*b*).

Having found that the visual system does indeed take short cuts to detect correspondence between images of a single object, we wondered what strategy the system would adopt when faced with many objects in apparent motion. Would it analyze each object independently or would it again take short cuts? Our studies suggest that the visual system tends economically to perceive all objects in a field as moving in the same way unless there are unambiguous cues to the contrary. Gestalt psychologists would call this a tendency to see "global field effects."

In two related experiments we rapidly and simultaneously displayed many bistable quartets, each of which could be perceived to be in vertical or horizontal oscillation. One experiment had the quartets in three neat rows, whereas the second experiment presented the quartets more randomly. We found that observers perceived all the quartets in each experiment as locking together so that they all had the same axis of motion (see Figure 9.12). If the visual system did not prefer to see an entire field behave uniformly, and if it processed each quartet independently, our views would have seen a mixture of horizontally and vertically oscillating dots.

The unified perception of the clustered quartets suggests that field effects may often be the result of generalizing from a particular instance. That is, the motion seen in one region of a visual field may be significantly influenced by such contextural cues as motion perceived in another part of the field. One way to test this is to cause a bistable quartet to take a "random walk" across the screen (see Figure 9.13). After showing three of four cycles of alternat-

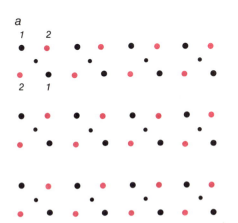 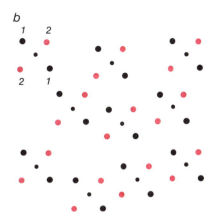

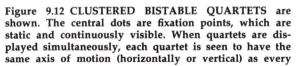

Figure 9.12 CLUSTERED BISTABLE QUARTETS are shown. The central dots are fixation points, which are static and continuously visible. When quartets are displayed simultaneously, each quartet is seen to have the same axis of motion (horizontally or vertical) as every other one, regardless of whether the quartets are arranged in regular rows (*a*) or are scattered randomly (*b*). This finding suggests that, in the absence of unambiguous cues to the contrary, the visual system tends to perceive all objects in a given field as moving in the same way.

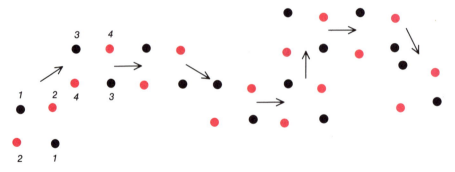

Figure 9.13 SEVEN QUARTETS that are displayed to subjects sequentially are presented here simultaneously. Arrows indicate the direction of movement from one bistable quartet to the next and numbers indicate the order of presentation of the dots. The dots in color are the ones flashed second in each quartet. Once viewers are the first quartet as having a vertical or a horizontal axis of motion, they almost always see the same axis in quartets presented later and perceive the quartets to be just a single quartet "walking" across the display screen.

ing dots in one bistable quartet, we switched off the display for about half a second before making it reappear elsewhere on the screen. Each of six individuals who viewed the display reported that the motion axis always remained the same even when the square moved to a new location. Once any particular motion axis was seen, the perception apparently acted as a template that created an enduring tendency to perceive similar motion in all other regions.

We recognized that subjects may have interpreted the four-dot display as a single object moving through space. To simplify the test of field effects further, one of us (Ramachandran, with his student Victor Inada) alternated images of eight randomly positioned dots with a set of identical dots shifted to the right (see Figure 9.14). Next we masked one of the dots in the second image. Normally when viewers are shown a single dot that is flashed on and off next to an apparent occluder, they see no oscillation. In the context of an array of oscillating dots, however, the perception changed: viewers saw the unpaired dot as oscillating horizontally behind the occluder. They saw what we call entrained motion; that is, motion in one part of the field caused the viewer to see the identical axis of motion in all other parts of the visual field. (The presence of the occluder strengthened the illusion, but the solitary dot also oscillated weakly when no occluder was shown.)

Our evidence indicates that in perceiving motion a viewer's visual system rapidly extracts sa-

lient features and applies built-in laws of motion when processing the features. It also responds to contextual clues in the rest of the field. Of course, even if one believes in the existence of such mechanisms and rejects the concept of laborious point-to-point matchings, an obvious—and much debated—question remains: How does the visual system apply all these strategies? Does it have neurons that are "hard-wired" with the strategies from birth? Or does the perception of motion require some higher level of cognition?

As we mentioned above, the experiments described in this chapter were designed to eliminate the effects of high-level cognition; specifically, we flashed images at speeds too rapid to allow the brain to make thoughtful decisions about what it was seeing. Our results therefore suggest that low-level processes can, on their own, control the perception of apparent motion during the early stages of visual processing.

Some other evidence also favors this notion over theories requiring the participation of intellect in early, as well as late, stages of motion perception. For instance, an illusion can be seen even when an individual knows an image is an illusion. Neurobiological evidence has been adduced in the past decade by David H. Hubel and Margaret S. Livingstone of the Harvard Medical School, by David C. Van Essen and John M. Allman of the California Institute of Technology and by Semir Zeki of University College London. They have found in monkeys that nerve cells sensitive to the motion of images with low spatial frequencies are distinct from the cells that are sensitive to color, line terminations, angles

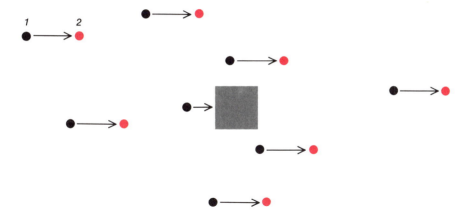

Figure 9.14 RANDOMLY PLACED DOTS are the basis of an illusion. The display results in entrained motion, in which motion seen in part of a field controls the motion seen elsewhere. In a continuous cycle, eight scattered dots (*black*) are flashed on the screen and are then replaced by eight identical dots (*color*) shifted to the right. Viewers see the dots move horizontally (*arrow*). When one dot in the second image is replaced with a patch on the display screen (*square*), as is shown here, the partner of the eliminated dot appears to move behind the patch as though entrained by the motion in the field.

and other sharp features. This is consistent with our finding that the brain's motion-detecting system pairs off objects sharing low spatial frequencies faster than it pairs off objects sharing sharp features, and it suggests that neuronal activity may be sufficient to account for the initial detection of correspondence by the viewer.

The cellular events that mediate early visual processing in human beings are still very much a mystery, but in time the neurobiological approach should combine with the psychological to elucidate the processes by which the visual system detects correspondence. Our findings suggest, meanwhile, that new advances in the construction of motion-detecting vision machines might be made if investigators who design those machines would attempt to substitute the tricks we have described here for the point-to-point schemes that are currently in vogue.

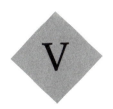

ILLUSORY PHENOMENA

. . .

Subjective Contours

Certain combinations of incomplete figures give rise to clearly visible contours even when the contours do not actually exist. It appears that such contours are supplied by the visual system.

· · ·

Gaetano Kanizsa
April, 1976

If we examine the conditions that give rise to visible contours, we usually find that a contour is perceived when there is a jump in the stimulation between adjacent areas. The jump may be due to a difference in brightness or a difference in color. There are conditions, however, that cause us to perceive contours in visual areas that are completely homogeneous. For example, in Figure 10.1 the solid triangles in the center of each figure appear to have well-defined contours, but close examination of the contours where they cross an open area reveals that they have no physical basis. If you fix your gaze on one of these contours, it disappears, yet if you direct your gaze to the entire figure, the contours appear to be real.

The phenomenon of contours that appear in the absence of physical gradients has aroused considerable interest among psychologists on both the experimental and the theoretical level. A number of variants of the effect have been discovered, and several explanations have been proposed for it. Here I shall describe some of the more interesting properties of the effect and examine some of the attempted explanations. First, however, let us consider a related visual phenomenon: the phenomenon of virtual lines.

When we view three dots that are equidistant from one another and are not in a straight line, the visual system spontaneously organizes the dots into a triangle. In addition the three dots appear to be connected by three straight lines. These lines are called virtual, and although they are not actually seen, they are a real presence in our visual experience. They are far more compelling than other connecting lines that can be imagined. For example, the three dots could just as readily be points on a circle, but the curved connecting lines of the circle are more difficult to "see" than the straight lines of the triangle.

Because virtual lines are only phenomenally present and do not have a sensory modality, one may speak of them as being "amodal." Another kind of amodal contour is found in partially hidden figures (see Figure 10.2). Consider a black rectangle that has a gray ring behind it and a colored ring in front of it. Although the missing contours of the rectangle are not actually seen, they nonetheless have a strong phenomenal presence. If the two rings in the illustration are now made black, a new effect results. Both black rings complete themselves behind the black rectangle in an amodal manner, but the contours of the rectangle are visible in their

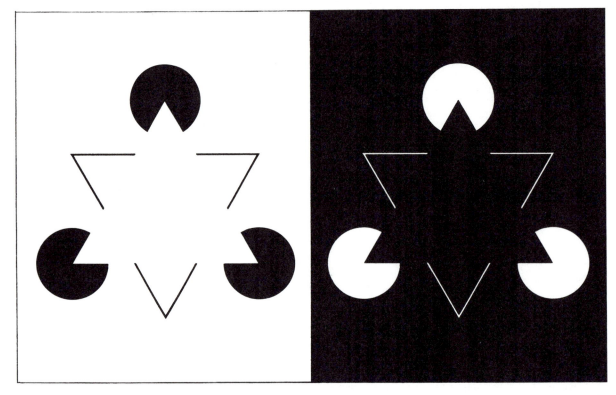

Figure 10.1 TWO SUBJECTIVE TRIANGLES, one whiter than white and the other blacker than black, appear to have distinct contours, but when the contours are examined closely, they disappear. The contours are subjective and have no physical reality. The region bounded by the subjective contours appears to be more intense than the background even though the color of the inner and the outer regions is identical.

entirety. Even in the homogeneous black regions where the rings overlap, the contours of the rectangle are visible. In other words, the contours have acquired a visual modality.

This "modal" presence is also found in the contours of the central triangles in Figure 10.1. Since those contours appear in the absence of the gradients that normally produce modal, or visible, contours, the situation is clearly anomalous. For that reason I prefer to call such contours anomalous contours. In order to emphasize the fact that the contours have no physical basis over most of their length, other investigators have called them subjective contours. They are also known as illusory contours. Whatever term is used, the phenomenon is the same.

W hat factors are involved in the formation of subjective contours? Analysis of many exam-

ples of the phenomenon yields the following common characteristics. First, the region that is bounded by the subjective contours appears to be brighter than the background, even though the visual stimulation provided by both regions is exactly the same. Second, the region within the subjective contours appears as an opaque surface that is superposed on the other figures in the illustration.

The subjective contours we have considered up to this point have all been straight lines. Is it possible to create curved subjective contours? As Figures 10.3 and 10.4 demonstrate, there are a variety of ways for generating such subjective contours. Indeed, even amorphous subjective figures can be created.

The strength of the phenomenon of subjective contours can be measured in part by determining the resistance such contours show to interference by real lines. When a real line intersects a subjective

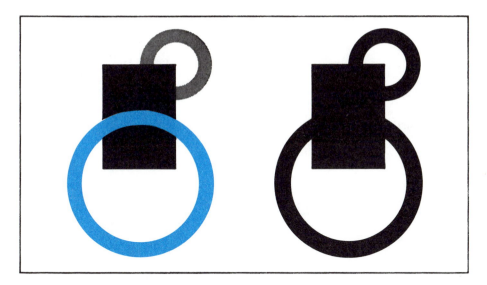

Figure 10.2 AMODAL AND MODAL CONTOURS are found in overlapping figures. Amodal contours are not actually seen, but they have a strong phenomenal presence. For example, the missing contours of the black rectangle complete themselves behind the colored ring in an amodal manner. Modal contours, on the other hand, appear to be visible. For example, the contours of the rectangle at the right are visible even in the regions where they overlap the black rings.

contour, the contour in that region disappears, indicating that it has a relatively low degree of resistance to interference. On the other hand, the opaque subjective surface displays surprising resistance: it appears to pass under lines that intersect it (see Figure 10.5). The subjective surface also displays strong resistance to interference within its borders. If large dark spots are placed inside the borders, the spots do not become part of the background but rather appear to be on the subjective surface. What

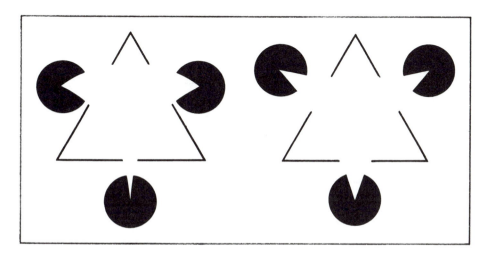

Figure 10.3 CURVED SUBJECTIVE CONTOURS are created by sectors with curved angles (*left*). Sectors with straight angles can create curved contours if angles are not aligned with one another.

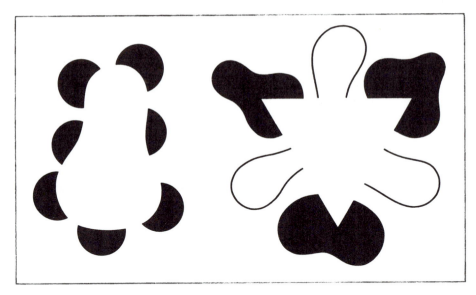

Figure 10.4 GEOMETRIC REGULARITY is not a necessary condition for the formation of subjective surfaces and contours. Amorphous shapes are possible and irregular figures can generate contours.

happens when the background, instead of being homogeneous, has a texture? It turns out that a texture does not impede the formation of subjective contours or surfaces (see Figure 10.5, right).

A number of optical illusions are produced by the reciprocal action between lines and surfaces. These optical illusions offer an opportunity to ascertain whether subjective contours and shapes have the same functional effects as objective, or real, contours and shapes. In many instances subjective contours and shapes are able to duplicate the illusion created by objective ones. As Figure 10.6 demon-

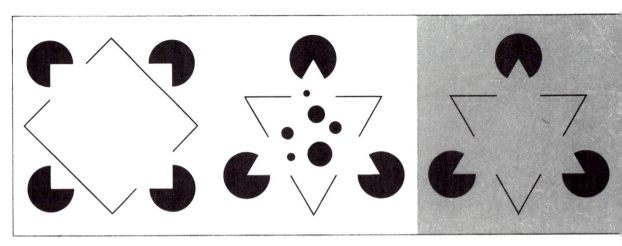

Figure 10.5 RESISTANCE TO INTERFERENCE is a measure of the perceptual strength of subjective surfaces. A subjective surface appears to pass under lines that intersect with it (*left*), but subjective contours are destroyed by the line. Spots inside the borders of the subjective surface become part of it (*middle*). The formation of subjective contours or surfaces is not impeded by the presence of a texture (*right*).

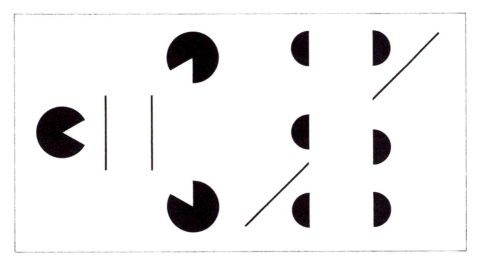

Figure 10.6 OPTICAL ILLUSIONS show that subjective contours have the same functional effects as real contours. In the Ponzo illusion (*left*), although both vertical lines are the same length, the effect of the subjective triangle is to make the line at the left appear to be longer. In the Poggendorf illusion the subjective surface gives rise to an apparent displacement of the slanted line.

strates, subjective contours and surfaces will interact with physically real lines to give rise to familiar optical illusions.

As we have seen, one of the characteristics of subjective surfaces is that they appear to be superposed on the other figures in the illustration. We have also seen that the subjective surface appears to be opaque. It is not difficult, however, to produce transparent subjective surfaces with distinct subjective contours (see Figure 10.7).

In most of the situations we have been examining the subjective surface appears to be brighter than

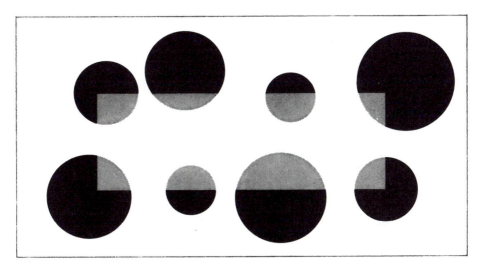

Figure 10.7 TRANSPARENT SUBJECTIVE SURFACES, as well as opaque ones, can be produced. The transparent surface, with clearly visible contours, seems to lie in a plane in front of black disks.

the background, even though the two regions are identical in brightness and color. It is possible that the brightness of the subjective surface is due to contrast enhancement. Such enhancement is generally found when a light surface is adjacent to one dark surface or more. The intensity of the effect depends on the extent of the dark surface. Although the brightness-contrast effect may play a role in creating subjective surfaces, it is not a necessary condition for the formation of such surfaces or contours. This is readily demonstrated in Figure 10.8, where a substantial reduction in the amount of black does not diminish the effect. A decisive item of evidence that contrast is not necessary for the formation of a subjective contour is presented in Figure 10.9. In this figure there are no differences in brightness that could be attributed to contrast, yet a curved subjective contour between the line segments is clearly visible.

It has been suggested by some investigators that subjective contours can be explained in terms of the partial activation of contour-detector cells in the visual system. According to this hypothesis, the short line segments in the visual stimulus activate some of the contour detectors, and signals from the activated detectors are interpreted as being a stimulus from a continuous line. The hypothesis does not stand up to careful examination, however. In many cases a subjective contour does not continue in the same direction as the stimulus line segments. More-

over, line segments are not necessary for the generation of subjective contours. In some instances the line segments can be replaced by dots and subjective contours will still be perceived (see Figure 10.9, right).

There is one condition, I have found, that is always present in the formation of subjective contours. That condition is the presence in the visual field of certain elements that are incomplete, which on completion are transformed into simpler stable and regular figures. For example, it could be said that the figure at the left in Figure 10.1 consists of three black sectors and three angles. Each of these figural elements is incomplete in some way. Most observers, however, report that they see a white triangle covering three black disks and another triangle with a black border. This perceptual organization has obvious advantages from the standpoint of simplicity and stability. The three angles become a triangle, a stabler and more balanced figure. The three circular sectors acquire completeness and regularity by becoming disks. In order for this perceptual organization to materialize, however, the white area in the center must be seen as an opaque triangle that is superposed on the other figures. And since the triangle must have a border, the necessary contours are supplied by the visual system. The contours are therefore the result of perceiving a surface and not vice versa. The subjective surface in turn is generated by the tendency of the visual system to complete certain figural elements.

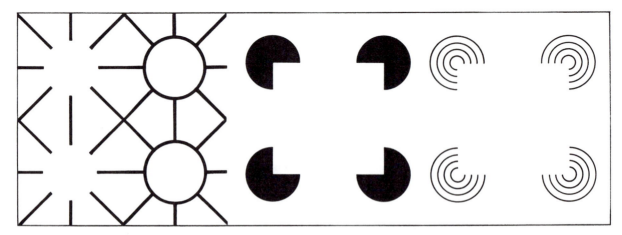

Figure 10.8 ENHANCED BRIGHTNESS of subjective surfaces is not due to contrast. If contrast were a primary condition of the effect, the black-ringed circles should ap- pear to be brighter than the subjective circles (*left*). Reducing amount of black does not diminish the effect (*right*).

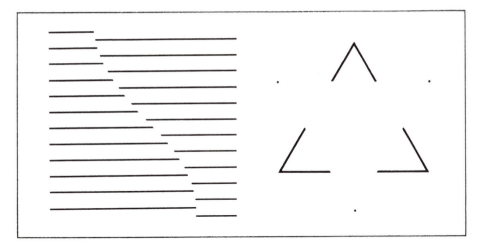

Figure 10.9 CONTOUR-DETECTOR HYPOTHESIS states that subjective contours are generated by partial activation of contour detectors in the visual system by short line segments in the stimulus. Subjective contours, however, can have an orientation completely different from that of the line segments (*left*). Furthermore, line segments are not necessary for generation of subjective contours (*right*). Curved subjective contour formed by line segments also demonstrates that differences in brightness due to contrast are not needed for formation of subjective contours.

If these assertions are correct, we should be able to demonstrate that subjective contours and shapes will not be perceived when the visual field does not contain incomplete figural elements. Since figures with open borders tend to appear incomplete, it is not difficult to create subjective contours with them. If we close the borders on these figures and make no other changes, the subjective contours disappear (see Figure 10.10)

The following, I believe, offers further confirma-

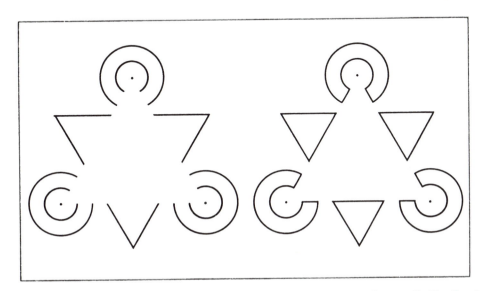

Figure 10.10 FIGURES WITH OPEN BORDERS appear to be incomplete. In order to complete the figures the visual system superposes an opaque surface that fills the gaps in the figures. Because the surface must have borders the necessary contours are also supplied by the visual system. If borders of figures are closed, there is no further need for completion and contours disappear.

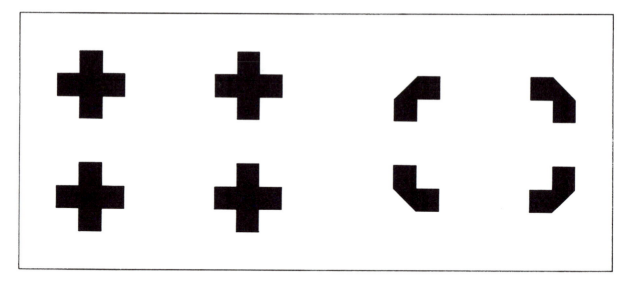

Figure 10.11 COMPLETE FIGURES do not generate subjective surfaces. Although crosses provide outlines of a rectangle, the rectangle is not perceived as a surface. When crosses are cut in half, a subjective rectangle is perceived and the half crosses are now seen as mutilated hexagons.

tion of the completion hypothesis. At the left in Figure 10.11, there are four black crosses on a white field. In spite of the fact that the crosses provide the outlines of a rectangle in the central region, we do not perceive the rectangle as a subjective surface. The reason is that the crosses are balanced and self-sufficient figures and do not require completion. When the crosses are cut in half, however, a subjective surface appears in the central area. The half crosses are in this case more likely to be seen as mutilated hexagons.

We have seen that irregularly shaped subjective

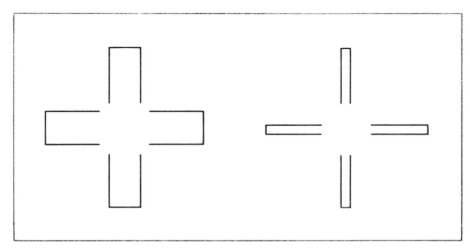

Figure 10.12 INCOMPLETE CROSS (*left*) gives rise to the unusual phenomenon of subjective angles. The angles are formed by the contours of the subjective square that covers central portion of the cross. Rectangular shape of the sub- jective surface is attributed to the resistance of arms of cross to invasion by the surface. If arms of cross are narrowed, circular subjective surface results.

figures can be produced. In most of my examples the incomplete figures I have used to create subjective contours have been regular and symmetrical. Although geometric figures may enhance the effect, however, they are by no means necessary (see Figure 10.4).

Finally, is it possible to generate subjective contours that meet and form a subjective angle? Paolo Sambin of the University of Padua found that an incomplete cross gives rise to such an effect (see Figure 10.12). According to Sambin, the rectangular shape of the subjective surface that is perceived is produced by the resistance of the arms of the cross to invasion by the subjective surface. Without such resistance the subjective contour would assume the shape of a circle. The validity of his hypothesis can be demonstrated by narrowing the arms of the cross to the point where the invasion of the internal area is minimal. Under those conditions the subjective surface that is perceived has the form of a circle.

A nother example of contour perception in the absence of brightness gradients is found in the random-dot stereograms created by Bela Julesz at Bell Laboratories. These stereograms do not reveal any contours when they are viewed monocularly, but when they are viewed with a stereoscope, they combine to form three-dimensional shapes and contours. Stanley Coren, then at the New School for Social Research, has advanced the hypothesis that the perceptual mechanism giving rise to subjective contours and shapes is the same as the mechanism giving rise to three-dimensional depth perception. (Julesz is currently at Rutgers University and Coren is at the University of British Columbia, Vancouver.)

Since the formation of subjective contours is usually connected with the generation of surfaces and their stratification, or apparent layering, the line of reasoning proposed by Coren may be valid. On the other hand, in all the cases that we have examined stratification depends on the completion of some figural elements. When there is no need for completion, stratification does not occur and there are no subjective contours. Once more the primary factor seems to be the tendency to completion. Stratification seems to arise as a function of this completion.

Geometrical Illusions

In these classic figures of psychology lines appear different from the way they really are. The effects appear to be related to clues to the size of objects in the three-dimensional world.

• • •

Barbara Gillam
January, 1980

Geometrical illusions are line figures in which the length, orientation, curvature or direction of lines is wrongly perceived. For example, in certain figures two lines of equal length appear to differ in length. Why does this happen? In normal three-dimensional viewing two lines of unequal length at different distances from the observer can cast on the retina images of equal size, but the lines are not perceived as being equal because the visual system takes into account the fact that they lie at different distances. The lines appear to have the lengths they actually have in the three-dimensional world because the perceptual mechanism known as size constancy seems to compensate for the difference in distance by making the far line appear to be larger and the near line appear to be smaller. It has been suggested that size constancy is responsible for geometrical illusions. In other words, if the visual system processed the lines of a geometric figure as if they were at different distances, then the result would be an illusion.

Attractive as this explanation of illusions may be, it is not correct because in most illusory line figures there is no depth, either real or apparent. It has nonetheless seemed to several investigators, including me, that some process contributing to accurate perceptions of the three-dimensional world might give rise to illusions in two-dimensional figures. My own finding is that geometrical illusions depend not on apparent depth but on clues to the scale and size of objects in the visible world, clues such as linear perspective and foreshortening. I shall be returning to this distinction between apparent depth and perspective clues in somewhat greater detail.

Most of the more than 200 geometric illusions that have been recorded by investigators were discovered in the second half of the 19th century. Some of the best-known illusions are shown in Figure 11.1 In the Müller-Lyer figure the two lines, one

Figure 11.1 NINE GEOMETRICAL ILLUSIONS are presented. In the upside-down T figure the vertical line and the horizontal line are the same length. In the Lipps figure the oblique lines in the middle are parallel. In both the Ponzo figure and the Müller-Lyer figure the horizontal lines are equal in length. In the Judd figure the dot is at the midpoint of the horizontal line. In the Poggendorff figure the oblique lines are collinear. In the Zöllner figure the oblique lines are parallel. In the Titchener figure the two inner circles are the same size. In the Delboeuf figure the outer circle on the left is the same size as the inner circle on the right.

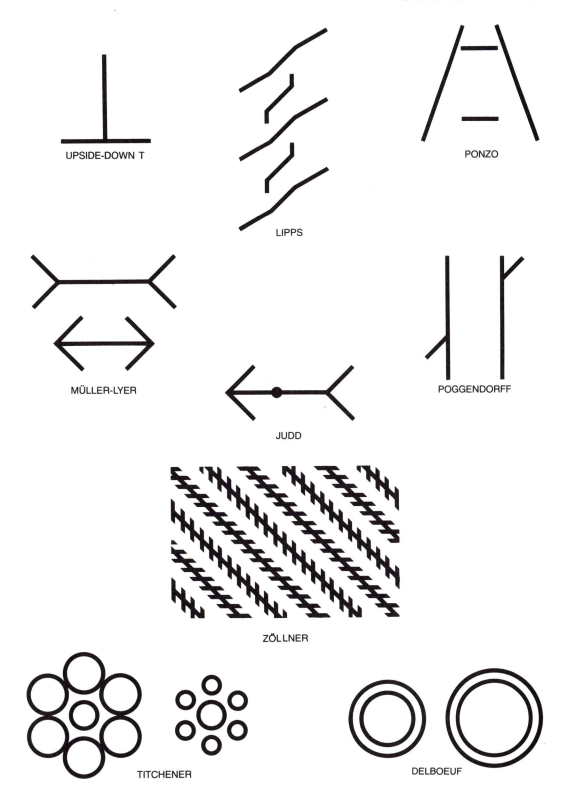

UPSIDE-DOWN T

LIPPS

PONZO

MÜLLER-LYER

JUDD

POGGENDORFF

ZÖLLNER

TITCHENER

DELBOEUF

with outward-pointing arrowheads at the ends and the other with inward-pointing arrowheads, are actually the same length. In the Ponzo figure the horizontal lines are also the same length. In both the Zöllner and Lipps figures the oblique lines are parallel. In the Titchener figure the two inner circles are the same size. In the Delboeuf figure the outer circle on the left is the same size as the inner circle on the right. In the Poggendorff figure the oblique lines are collinear. In the upside-down T the horizontal and vertical lines are the same length. And in the Judd figure the dot is at the middle of the horizontal line.

Each of these illusions has traditionally been thought to consist of two parts: an "inducing" component that does the distorting and a "test" component that is distorted. For example, in the Müller-

Lyer figure the arrowheads are the inducing component and the horizontal lines are the test component, and in the Poggendorff figure the parallel lines are the inducing component and the oblique lines are the text component. This division can, however, oversimplify what is going on. The distortion of the test component is sometimes only the most obvious manifestation of a host of misperceptions that involve the inducing component as well (see Figure 11.2)

In the 100 years that geometrical illusions have been studied many different explanations for them have been advanced. The most compelling of these explanations agree on three fundamental points. First, the illusions are not conceptual but

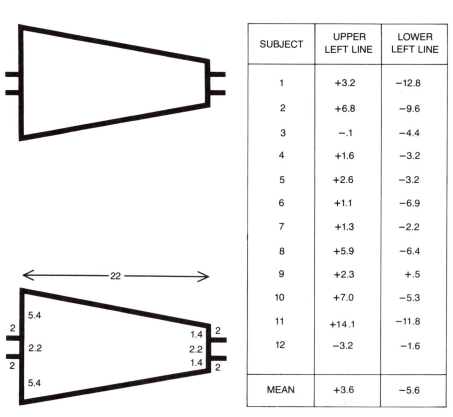

SUBJECT	UPPER LEFT LINE	LOWER LEFT LINE
1	+3.2	−12.8
2	+6.8	−9.6
3	−.1	−4.4
4	+1.6	−3.2
5	+2.6	−3.2
6	+1.1	−6.9
7	+1.3	−2.2
8	+5.9	−6.4
9	+2.3	+.5
10	+7.0	−5.3
11	+14.1	−11.8
12	−3.2	−1.6
MEAN	+3.6	−5.6

Figure 11.2 IN VARIATION OF THE PONZO ILLUSION (*top left*) collinear line segments seem to be displaced. The author asked 12 subjects how much each line at the left should be adjusted to make it collinear with the corresponding line at the right. For the figure at the bottom left (dimensions in centimeters), the subjects' adjustments are tabulated in millimeters at the right. In the normal Ponzo illusion in Figure 11.1, the apparent length of the upper line is distorted toward the surround (assimilation), whereas the apparent length of the lower line is distorted away from the surround (contrast). Yet there is more to the illusion. The figure at the top left shows that the Ponzo configuration affects not only length of lines placed in it but also alignment of lines attached to its end.

perceptual; knowing that a particular effect is illusory does not diminish the strength of the illusion, although most of the illusions are drastically reduced when the figure is viewed repeatedly over a short period of time. Second, the illusions do not originate in the retina; they emerge at almost full strength when the inducing component is presented to one eye and the test component is presented to the other, and so they must originate at a point in the visual system beyond the lateral geniculate nucleus of the brain, where the inputs from the two eyes first come together. Third, illusions do not result from the movements of the eye; experiments show that the illusions, usually of full magnitude, emerge when a figure is exposed too briefly for the eye to scan it or when the retinal image of the figure is artificially stabilized by a special apparatus that causes the image to remain still on the retina even as the eye moves back and forth.

Explanations of illusions fall into four main categories: classification theories, activity theories, physiological theories and functional theories. The theories are not necessarily mutually exclusive; in some cases they might emphasize different aspects of the same process. The first of these categories is the least ambitious. The classification theories point to common properties among a variety of illusory figures. What the figures have in common suggests the presence of an underlying perceptual process. Neither the mechanism nor the function of such a process is addressed by the classification theories. The illusions are attributed to contrast when they are characterized by a perceptual exaggeration of the degree to which the test component differs from the inducing component in a prevailing quality such as size or orientation. The Titchener illusion is an example of size contrast, whereas the Zöllner illusion is one of orientation contrast, or more specifically of angle contrast.

The illusions are attributed to assimilation or confusion when they are characterized by a perceptual underestimation of the degree to which the test component differs from the inducing component. In other words, the test element is distorted in the same direction as a prevailing quality of the inducing element. The Müller-Lyer illusion is an example of size or position assimilation because the horizontal lines are lengthened in the direction of the arrowheads. The Lipps illusion is an example of orientation assimilation because the orientation of each parallel line is perceptually shifted toward the orientation of its neighbors. A single illusion can incorporate both contrast and assimilation. In the Ponzo illusion the apparent length of the upper line is distorted toward the surround (assimilation), whereas the apparent length of the lower line is distorted away from the surround (contrast).

This classification scheme has done little more than help to bring order to the large number of illusions. It does suggest, however, that the processes could have something in common with those of brightness perception, which exhibits both contrast and assimilation with respect to the brightness of neighboring areas in a scene. Apart from the classification scheme's lack of explanatory power, it is limited by the fact that it does not apply to some important illusions, for example the Poggendorff figure and the upside-down T. Moreover, the lines that are assimilated in the Lipps figure are well within the orientation range of the lines that show contrast in the Zöllner figure.

The activity and physiological theories go beyond mere classification by asserting that illusions are incidental side effects or errors of normal visual perception. Activity theories attribute illusions to the responses an individual has to certain stimuli or prepares to have to them. The efferent-readiness theory, proposed by Leon Festinger at the New School for Social Research [Festinger died in 1989.], maintains that illusions develop because of the way the eye "gets ready" for saccadic movements. (As I have mentioned, experimental evidence rules out the eye movements themselves playing a role in the illusions, but that evidence does not rule out the possibility that the visual system's preparations for eye movements do play such a role.) According to this theory, people tend to look not at the entire figure but at the part of the figure that optimizes the number of details seen with high acuity. Festinger and his co-workers have found that when people try to fixate on the ends of a Müller-Lyer figure, they actually fixate within the arrowheads. According to Festinger, that has the effect of lengthening the line with the inward-pointing arrowheads and shortening the line with the outward-pointing ones.

It is known that the decrease in the strength of an illusion that comes with repeated exposure is accompanied by an increase in the accuracy of eye movements, but this correlation does not indicate whether or not the eye movements cause the illusions. Many other motor responses, such as directing a pointer at the illusion, might provide information about the perceptual error and thereby help to reduce the illusion in the same way that eye movements do. Inasmuch as the illusion would not be attributed to the intention to direct a pointer, it would be premature in the absence of other evidence to attribute the illusion to preparations for saccadic eye movements. Moreover, it is difficult to understand why inaccurate eye movements in the presence of angle and line intersections would not have been eliminated in the normal environment where such intersections are frequently encountered.

The physiological theories attribute illusions to the "hardware" of the visual system. Many of these theories are based on lateral inhibition, a neural process that serves to restrict the stimuli that can fire a cell in the visual cortex of the brain. According to these theories, the perceived orientation of a line is determined by the peak activity of orientation-detecting cells in the visual cortex, each of which is activated by line stimuli of a particular range of orientations. The introduction of a second line of a different but similar orientation gives rise to a somewhat different distribution of activity among the orientation-detecting cells, activity that either facilitates or inhibits the activity generated by the first line, thereby shifting the apparent orientation. On this view facilitation, which would result from very similar lines, would cause assimilation in the illusory figure, and inhibition, which would result from less similar lines, would cause contrast. The same view is supported by the experiments of Colin Blakemore and his co-workers at the University of Cambridge (see Figure 11.3). To explain size illusions a similar physiological theory has been proposed that is based on size-detecting cells in the visual cortex.

Physiological theories based on lateral inhibition are best able to handle angle-contrast illusions with multiple inducing lines, for example the Zöllner illusion, which exhibits assimilation at extremely small angles and contrast at larger angles. George Wallace and his co-workers at the University of Reading have found that the Zöllner illusion is enhanced by changes that should promote lateral inhibition, such as increasing either the brightness contrast or the number of inducing lines.

Most angle-contrast illusions persist when the test line is replaced by a set of dots or by a moving dot. Physiological theories based on lateral inhibition cannot explain this phenomenon because there is no actual test line to be inhibited. That may not be a problem, however, because little work has been done on whether the orientation-detecting cells might in fact respond selectively not only to a line but also to a row of dots or a moving dot.

Physiological theories based on lateral inhibition fall short for the simplest illusions involving angles. For example, in the Poggendorff figure the acute angles, which should show the greatest effect of lateral inhibition, contribute nothing to the illusion (see Figure 11.4). Another exception is the Müller-Lyer illusion, which no physiological theory has been able to explain. A comparison of the horizontal lines of the Müller-Lyer figure with a line lacking arrowheads reveals that the inward-pointing-arrowhead configuration (obtuse angles) contributes two or three times as much to the total illusion as the outward-pointing-arrowhead configuration (acute angles). No plausible arrangement of orientation-detecting cells could give rise to such lopsided contributions.

Another physiological theory, filter theory, is based on neural channels in the visual cortex that seem to be tuned not to line stimuli but to particular spatial frequencies of sinusoidal modulations of light, the spatial frequency being the number of modulations per unit of visual angle. Mathematicians have proved that any waveform, no matter how complicated, can be expressed as the sum of simple sinusoidal waveforms. In 1968 Fergus W. Campbell and John G. Robson of the University of Cambridge proposed that the visual system processes a waveform of light by breaking it down into its sinusoidal components. Since then much psychophysical and physiological evidence has accumulated in support of this proposal, and it is now a cornerstone of visual theory.

Arthur Ginsberg of the U.S. Air Force attributes illusions to the responses of the neural channels that are tuned to low spatial frequencies. He has broken down the images of certain illusory figures into sinusoidal waveforms of different frequencies and amplitudes, eliminated the high-frequency waveforms and added back together the low-frequency ones. With the high-frequency waveforms filtered out the reconstructed image turns out to have properties that correspond to perceived distortions of the original figure. For example, in the reconstructed image of the outward-pointing-arrowhead configuration of the Müller-Lyer illusion the arrowheads and the shaft have merged to form a short blurred shaft, and in the reconstructed image of the inward-pointing-arrowhead configuration the arrowheads and

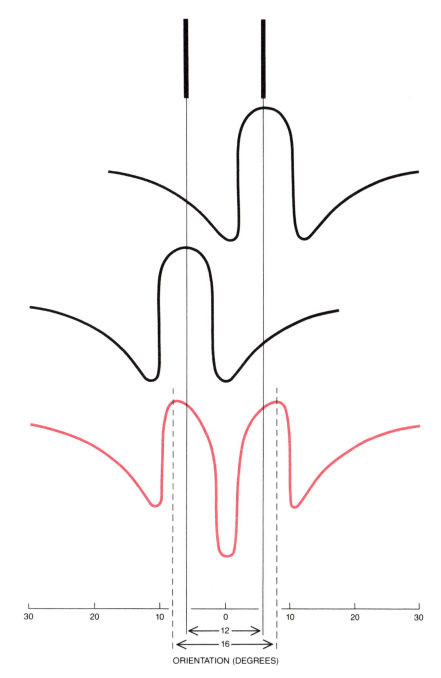

Figure 11.3 VISUAL RESPONSE TO LINE STIMULI is shown in a highly schematic way for two lines that differ in orientation by 12 degrees. Below each line is the distribution of orientation-detecting cells of the visual cortex that the line activates. The colored distribution shows what might happen if the two lines were presented simultaneously to the visual system. The sum of the individual distributions gives rise to the colored distribution in which the peaks of activity are slightly displaced from each other. This figure is based on the findings of Colin Blakemore, Roger H. S. Carpenter and their colleagues at the University of Cambridge.

the shaft have merged to form a long blurred shaft. The respective shortening and lengthening of the shaft is of course the substance of the illusion.

Ingenious as Ginsberg's work may be, there is little reason to believe that in arriving at size judg-

ments the visual system filters out the information provided by high-frequency waveforms. It would be odd (although not impossible) if the visual system judged the apparent size of a distinct line by the responses of neural channels in which the line was

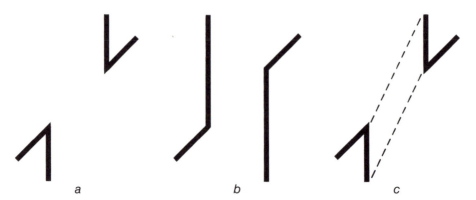

Figure 11.4 POGGENDORFF FIGURE is decomposed so that the illusory effects of the acute-angle components (*a*) can be distinguished from those of the obtuse-angle components (*b*). In *a* the illusion is zero or even slightly negative, the line at the right appearing to some people to be slightly lower than the one at the left. In *b* the illusion is strongly present. An illusion in *a* may be due to the visual system's processing *a* as if it were part of *c*, in which parallel lines form a receding place. In *c* the line at the right is in fact lower on the receding plane than the one at left.

indistinctly merged with its surround, particularly because such judgments would lead to gross perceptual errors.

A major drawback of both activity theories and physiological theories is that they cannot account for the decreases in the strength of illusions. The fact that by repeated exposure illusions can diminish almost to zero for as long as a period of days does not support theories that posit immutable physiological mechanisms. Only functional theories, which treat illusions not as errors but as essential processes of the visual system, begin to deal adequately with decreases in the strength of illusions.

Over the past century several investigators, including the 19th-century psychologist Armand Thiéry, Richard L. Gregory of the University of Bristol and Reinhardt Tausch of the University of Marburg, have shown that most illusory figures can be found in two-dimensional representations of three-dimensional scenes. What are called distortions or illusions in sketchy drawings promote accurate perception in the normal three-dimensional world and increase the realism of a picture. Consider Figure 11.5. One guitar looks longer than the other (the Ponzo illusion), the rear edge of the carpet looks shorter than its front-to-back dimension (the upside-down T), the molding looks too high to be collinear with the baseboard (the Poggendorff illusion) and the front edge of the carpet looks shorter

than the bottom edge of the back wall (the Müller-Lyer illusion with half of each arrowhead).

Although all these percepts are distortions compared with the picture plane or the retinal image, they would not normally be called illusions because they are not surprising. They reflect characteristics of the three-dimensional world represented in the picture plane. In normal three-dimensional viewing it is quite irrelevant whether or not a baseboard is retinally collinear with a molding and whether or not the edge of a door has the same length in the retinal image as the corner of a room. Such facts about the picture plane, which depend mostly on the viewing position of the observer, are not registered.

The main function of perception is to decode the transient retinal image in order to achieve constancy: the perception of the external world in terms of its stable and intrinsic characteristics. In the illustration of the room it is clear that the "distortions" are just instances of perception doing its job. If the contextual details that are necessary for a three-dimensional impression are eliminated, however, the same perceptual responses to the same configurations seem unjustified and are called illusions. Does this mean that illusions are only constancy responses (the decoding of perspective) operating in a context that is too minimal, since it lacks apparent depth, to give the distortions meaning? This view is appealingly parsimonious, but it goes against a

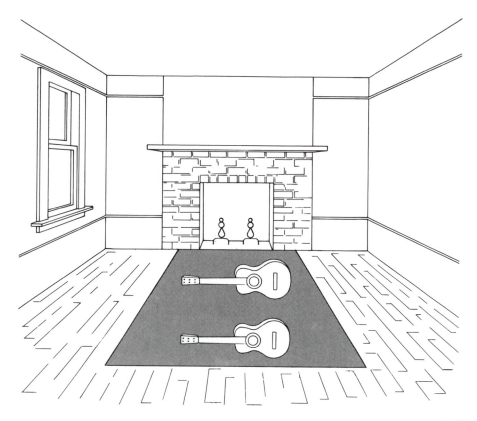

Figure 11.5 PICTURE OF A LIVING ROOM includes many well-known illusory configurations. One guitar looks longer than the other (Ponzo illusion), the rear edge of the carpet looks shorter than its front-to-back dimension (upside-down-T illusion), the molding looks too high to be collinear with the baseboard (Poggendorff illusion) and the front edge of the carpet looks shorter than the bottom edge of the back wall (Müller-Lyer illusion with half of each arrowhead).

strong tradition in psychology that constancy responses are triggered by apparent depth.

There are a number of reasons to doubt that a depth response always underlines constancy scaling. J. J. Gibson of Cornell University has pointed out that gradients in the apparent compression of objects and textures by perspective provide information about the size and shape of objects. The size of an object can often be judged by the ratio of its width to the width of the background. Consider railroad tracks receding into the distance. Since the viewer knows that the distant railroad ties are as large as the close ones, an object spanning the rails in the distance is perceived as being the same size as an object spanning the rails in the foreground, in spite of the fact that the sizes of the objects' retinal images are quite different.

Conclusive evidence for a size-constancy process that is not secondary to perceived depth comes from my own work with backgrounds in which equivalent depths are represented by different types of perspective (see Figures 11.6 and 11.7). In effect I was able to separate the response to depth from the response to perspective. I investigated two kinds of background drawing. In the first kind, based on the receding oblique lines of the Ponzo figure, the horizontal dimensions are increasingly compressed toward the "far" end, or top, of the drawing (the distortion known as linear perspective). In the second drawing, based on horizontal parallel lines that get closer to one another toward the top of the drawing, the vertical dimensions are increasingly compressed (the distortion known as foreshortening).

Next I put test lines at various orientations on the

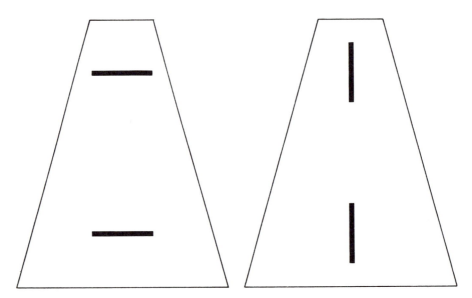

Figure 11.6 LINEAR PERSPECTIVE, the compression of horizontal dimensions toward the top of a drawing, is achieved by the receding oblique lines of the Ponzo figure. The horizontal test lines (*left*) are the same length, but the upper line appears to be longer because of linear perspective. There is no illusion for vertical test lines (*right*). This means that here the perception of size depends not on depth, which would increase the length of all the test lines regardless of their orientation, but on perspective, which affects only lines for which the background shows a scale of size.

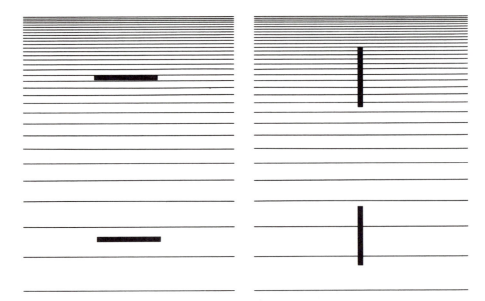

Figure 11.7 FORESHORTENING, the compression of vertical dimensions toward the top of a drawing, is achieved by parallel horizontal lines that get closer to one another toward the top of the drawing. The vertical test lines (*right*) are the same length, but the upper one seems longer because of foreshortening. There is no illusion for the horizontal test lines (*left*). This result confirms that the perception of size here does not depend on depth, which would lengthen horizontal lines as well as vertical ones. Perception of size seems to depend on the perspective scale of size.

two kinds of background. I found that the perceptual lengthening of lines put at the top with respect to lines put at the "near" end, or bottom, occurred only when the test lines were oriented along the compressed dimensions. There was no illusion for test lines at orientations for which the background drawing did not provide a scale of size. In other words, a linear-perspective scale does not affect the apparent length of lines along the dimension subject to foreshortening. This result constitutes compelling evidence for a perceptual mechanism promoting size constancy that is based on the scale itself and not on a depth response to the scale, which would lengthen any apparently distant lines regardless of their orientation.

This is not to deny that apparent distance can influence size perception. Experiments have demonstrated that changes in perceived size and shape accompany depth reversal in ambiguous figures. The fact that perceived size and shape can be primary responses and yet can still be influenced by apparent depth is not surprising when one considers that depth perception itself can be influenced by apparent size and shape. An example is the well-known moon illusion. When the moon is near the horizon, it looks larger than it does high in the sky. As a result when it is near the horizon, it looks closer. Under normal circumstances primary and secondary ways of judging size and distance reinforce each other. My work shows, however, that the amount of information in a line drawing needed to trigger a primary process of size scaling is less than the amount needed to trigger a process of depth scaling. Gregory has suggested that this result may be due to a perceptual conflict between the drawing's representing objects in depth and its actually being flat.

How well can a functional theory based not on apparent depth but on perspective explain illusions that do not have an interpretation as obvious in terms of perspective as the Ponzo illusion does? How does it explain the Müller-Lyer or the Poggendorff illusion? The resemblance between the Müller-Lyer figure and objects and scenes involving depth has been recognized since the 19th century. Most recently Gregory has pointed to the similarity between the two Müller-Lyer configurations and the corner of a building seen respectively from the inside and the outside. On the other hand, Tausch and other investigators, including me, have found that the Müller-Lyer illusion is close to being the

sum of the separate effects of the four individual oblique lines forming the arrowheads on the length of the horizontal line, effects that seem to be divorced from depth. Two lines that form acute angles are perceptually shortened, whereas two that form obtuse angles are lengthened. It is the distortion of these fundamental angle relations that must be understood in order to comprehend the Müller-Lyer illusions and other illusions in which angles influence perceived line length.

Do the lengthening of lines bounded by obtuse angles and the shortening of lines bounded by acute angles promote perceptual constancy? They do. An overwhelmingly large proportion of the obtuse and acute angles formed on the retina in the course of human visual experience are projections of right angles. A perceptual mechanism that lengthens horizontal lines bounded by obtuse angles and shortens horizontal lines bounded by acute angles would compensate for the differences in size created by perspective projection (see Figure 11.8).

The figure also shows that the process I have described would promote size and shape constancy regardless of whether the obtuse angles represent far corners and the acute angles near ones or the obtuse angles represent near corners and the acute angles far ones. It is therefore not surprising that the presence or absence of these distortions has nothing to do with depth. The parts of the perspective projection of a rectangle that form obtuse angles are always the most contracted and the parts that form acute angles are always the most expanded. The fact that the obtuse angles have a much larger effect in the Müller-Lyer illusion suggests that constancy scaling tends to equalize lengths by expanding the most contracted parts (bounded by obtuse angles) to match the rest of the projection rather than to diminish the more expanded parts (bounded by acute angles) to match the rest of the projection.

If contraction and expansion illusions serve to compensate for properties of the projection that are not properties of the scene that was projected, then the greater the distortions caused by perspective projection are, the greater is the illusion needed to compensate for the distortion. That is the case with the Müller-Lyer illusion, which gets stronger as the angles deviate more from right angles and as the arrowheads become larger. (There is a limit I cannot account for, however, on the effect the size of the arrowheads has on the magnitude of the illusion.)

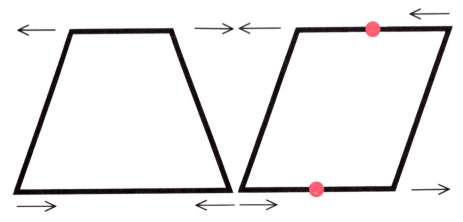

Figure 11.8 QUADRANGLES ON THE RETINA are usually the projections of rectangles in three-dimensional space. A perceptual mechanism that lengthens horizontal lines bounded by obtuse angles and shortens horizontal lines bounded by acute angles would compensate for the difference in size caused by perspective projection. The arrows indicate the direction of the perceptual expansion or contraction. The colored dots marked the midpoints of the horizontal lines of the quadrangle at the right. The midpoints appear to be too close to perceptually shortened ends.

I want to turn now to the Poggendorff illusion and discuss what it means in terms of perspective. The oblique lines of the Poggendorff figure do not seem to be significantly misaligned when they are viewed alone. Why does insertion of the vertical parallel lines disrupt the apparent alignment of the oblique lines to such a great degree? Although collinear lines in the three-dimensional world always project as collinear lines on the retina, noncollinear lines in the three-dimensional world can also project as collinear lines. I contend that the parallel lines of the Poggendorff figure, particularly the components forming obtuse angles, provide a context suggesting that the oblique lines do not represent collinear lines in three-dimensional space. As a result the oblique lines do not appear to be collinear. This is shown in Figure 11.10.

From the point of view of perspective, oblique lines represent receding horizontal lines. When two oblique lines are lined up, as they are in the Pog-

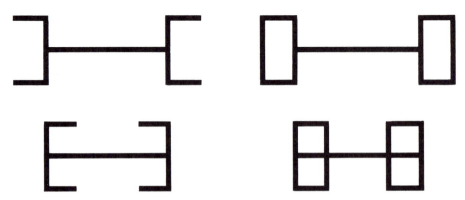

Figure 11.9 RECTANGULAR MÜELLER-LYER FIGURES (*left*) also create an illusion, although it is much weaker than the one created by the normal Müller-Lyer figures that are shown in Figure 11.1. The illusion gets quite strong when the appendages are closed up to form rectangles (*right*). No theory of geometrical illusions can account for this phenomenon.

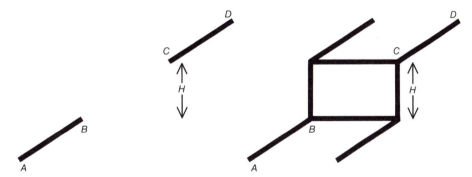

Figure 11.10 COLLINEAR LINES ON THE RETINA need not represent collinear lines in three-dimensional space. The ponts *B* and *C* could either represent an interruption in a continuous receding horizontal dimension (*left*), in which case the line *ABCD* would lie on one horizontal plane in three-dimensional space, or represent points separated horizontally and vertically (*right*), in which case *AB* and *CD* would lie on different horizontal planes and would therefore be noncollinear in three-dimensional space. The presence of parallel vertical lines in the Poggendorff figure favors the arrangement at the right, and so the visual system interprets the lines *AB* and *CD* as having different heights.

gendorff illusion, the conventions of perspective dictate that the space between them on the picture plane could represent one of two possible arrangements. The points *B* and *C* in the illustration could represent an interruption in a continuous receding horizontal dimension, in which case the line *ABCD* would lie on a single horizontal plane in three-dimensional space. The other possibility is that *B* and *C* represent points that are separated both horizontally and vertically, in which case *AB* and *BC* would lie on different horizontal planes and would therefore be noncollinear in three-dimensional space.

Visual processing favors the noncollinear arrangement when details placed within the gap *BC* are consistent with equidistance rather than with a depth difference for *B* and *C*. The parallel lines of the Poggendorff figure are particularly effective in this regard because they place *B* and *C* on a plane seen head on. What actually seems to happen is that the context changes the arrangement from one in which *AB*, *BC* and *CD* are each seen as having less slope than they do on the picture plane, because they all represent horizontal lines, to one in which the apparent slopes of *AB* and *CD* remain the same, because they continue to represent horizontal lines, whereas the apparent slope of *BC* increases, because it no longer represents a horizontal line. The result is a disruption of perceived collinearity. This explanation is supported experimentally by the work of

Ross H. Day and R. G. Dickinson of Monash University in Australia, who asked experimental subjects to estimate the slopes of *AB*, *BC* and *CD* in the Poggendorff figure.

An consequence of my explanation of the Poggendorff figure is that the illusion should be greatly reduced if the length of the parallel lines is changed so that they outline not a plane seen head on but an appropriately receding plane, in which case *AB*, *BC* and *CD* are collinear in three-dimensional space. This change can be achieved by making the ends of the parallel lines and the oblique lines converge on a single vanishing point. When the vanishing point is clearly defined, the magnitude of the illusion is reduced by half. This provides strong evidence that the context relevant to the three-dimensional layout represented by two-dimensional lines strongly influences the perceived collinearity (see Figure 11.11).

The evaluation of a functional theory based on perspective decoding is hampered by the fact that so little is known about perceptual responses to perspective, in spite of the fact that much of Western art has been based on perspective for 500 years. It is unlikely, however, that all illusions are the result of perspective decoding. For example, no obvious constancy function is served by illusions of orientation assimilation, such as the Lipps figure. Yet my functional theory, unlike the other theories, can handle

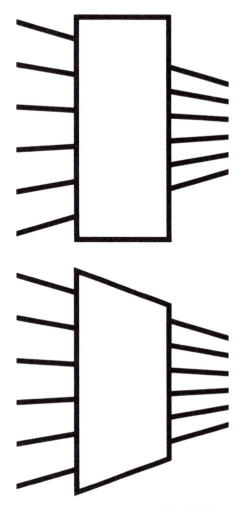

Figure 11.11 ORIENTATION OF THE PLANE strongly alters an illusion for a set of collinear oblique lines with a common vanishing point. The top lines, which interrupt a plane seen head on, appear to deviate more from being collinear than the bottom lines, which interrupt a receding place that has the same vanishing point as the lines. This provides evidence that the context relevant to the three-dimensional layout represented by lines in two dimensions strongly influences the perceived collinearity.

in a general way the maintenance of illusory responses under normal three-dimensional viewing conditions, where the responses are reinforced because they promote accurate perception, and the diminution of illusory responses under two-dimensional viewing conditions, where the responses are inhibited because they serve no function.

Work remains to be done on how the diminution is achieved and on what role eye movements play in the process. Stanley Coren of the University of British Columbia and Joan S. Girgus of Princeton University have proposed that illusions that strongly diminish in the course of repeated exposure have a considerable judgmental or learned component, whereas illusions that only weakly diminish, for example assimilation illusions such as the Delboeuf one, are chiefly built in. Although constancy responses are traditionally regarded as being based on learned algorithms, there is no reason some of the responses could not be built-in ones that evolved because they promoted constancy. In principle theories emphasizing function are not incompatible with theories emphasizing mechanism.

Functional theories based on perspective are supported to some degree by responses to geometrical illusions among peoples who do not live in a world dominated by rectangular rooms, buildings and cities. For such people the illusions tend to be not as strong as they are for people in our own kind of culture. Their response to the upside-down T illusion, on the other hand, which seems to depend not on the exposure to a rectangular environment but on the foreshortening of distant terrain, is not reduced. Striking as such results are, they should not be allowed to carry much theoretical weight until it is clear the people involved in the experiments have had the same understanding of what it is they are being asked to do as subjects in our own kind of culture. If such results hold up, however, they could significantly bolster the functional theories.

Perhaps the most serious challenge to functional theories, and for that matter to all theories of illusion relying on processes in the visual system, could come from investigations into the sense of touch. Experiments have revealed touch illusions that are analogous to optical ones when subjects ran their fingers over raised versions of well-known illusory figures. At this stage, however, the work is too tentative to establish any identity between misperceptions of touch and misperceptions of vision.

SECTION

PERCEPTION AND IMAGERY

. . .

Mental Imagery and the Visual System

What is the relation between mental imagery and visual perception? Recent work suggests the two share many of the same neural processes in the human visual system.

. . .

Ronald A. Finke
March, 1986

People often report that they can form mental images of an object that resemble the object's actual appearance. The act of constructing such images often produces visual sensations that seem quite realistic. Imagine, for example, that you are looking at an elephant. Does it have a curved trunk? What color are its tusks? How big are its eyes? Most people contend they attempt to answer such questions by "inspecting" a mental image in much the same way as they would inspect a real elephant.

These informal observations about imagery naturally lead one to consider the extent to which imagery and visual perception might be related. They suggest in particular that mental imagery may involve many of the same kinds of internal neural processes that underlie visual perception, a possibility that would have important theoretical and practical implications. If it could be established, for instance, that mental imagery shares with visual perception common neural mechanisms in the human visual system, one could begin to establish just how imagery may interact with visual perception. This would make it possible to explore the various ways imagery could function to facilitate, enhance or even substitute for visual perception, as

the art—by a blind woman—in Figure 12.1 suggests.

For the past 10 years my colleagues and I have been developing techniques for investigating the functional relation between mental imagery and visual perception. Because experimental subjects can often guess what ought to happen in an imagery experiment, we have striven to make our techniques precise enough to reveal subtle correspondences between imagery and perception. Our work has revealed that mental images display a much richer variety of visual properties than had been previously thought, but also that imagery differs from perception in certain respects.

Through introspection one can recognize that features of a mental image formed at a small size or a far distance are harder to distinguish than features of an image formed at a large size or a near distance. Try, for example, to imagine an ant on a newspaper several feet away and then on the tip of a toothpick directly in front of your eyes. You should be able to mentally "see" many more of the ant's features (such as its head and body segments) when you imagine it at close range.

Stephen M. Kosslyn of Harvard University ex-

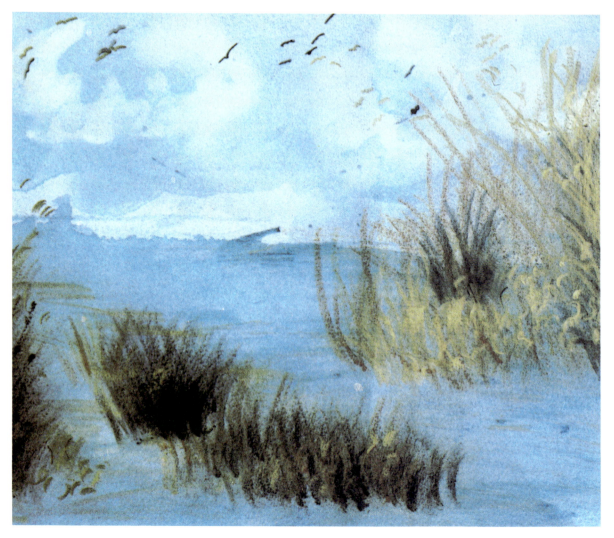

Figure 12.1 WATERCOLOR LANDSCAPE was painted by a blind Scotswoman who works from her mental images. The artist, Carolyn James, suffers from a particularly acute form of the eye disease known as retinitis pigmentosa. Now in her forties, she was registered blind at 21. To paint she lines up 24 watercolor jars in front of her in a memorized order. She moves from section to section on the paper, determining what she has just finished by detecting the moisture with her fingertips. Her watercolors are typically composed of six layers of paint.

plored this relation between image size and feature resolution by employing simple reaction-time techniques. He found that the features of an imagined animal, such as the eyes and ears of a cat, could be detected more quickly when subjects were instructed to fashion relatively large images or assume a relatively close vantage. The experiments were inspired by the common observation that features of real physical objects can be detected faster when they are viewed from a closer distance.

More recently Howard S. Kurtzman and I have done experiments at Cornell University to measure precisely how well the features of objects can be resolved, or distinguished, in imagery and in perception. We were particularly interested in how the size of the features, their spacing and their position in the visual field affected resolution, or the ability to distinguish among details. We predicted that across all these variations visual resolution in mental imagery should match the resolution in perception.

Resolution in visual perception falls off continually as one observes an object at locations progressively farther from the point of eye fixation. The amount of detail that can be distinguished is not the same in all directions, however. As a rule resolution decreases more slowly along the horizontal axis of the visual field than along the vertical axis, and more slowly below the point of fixation than above it. It is also known that bar gratings become harder to resolve as the gratings become increasingly finer —more precisely, as their fundamental spatial frequency increases.

Our method for measuring limits of resolution in mental imagery was based on certain techniques common to visual psychophysics. Initially we showed our subjects a flat disk whose upper half was filled with a series of vertical bars and whose lower half was filled with a series of horizontal bars. The bars in both gratings were the same width. We then instructed our subjects to form a mental image

of the disk and to project the image on the center of a screen directly in front of them (see Figure 12.2). On the screen eight lines extended radially out from the center. The subjects indicated how far they could look away from their images along each of the lines on the display before they could no longer tell the two halves of the imagined pattern apart. They reported that the gratings appeared fuzzy and indistinct as they were imagined farther into the visual periphery and then could no longer be distinguished beyond a certain point. For comparison, the same judgments were also obtained in a perception condition, in which the same disk was actually projected on the center of the screen in front of the subjects.

We repeated the experiment for each of three disks. The bar widths of the second disk were three times thinner than those of the first; those of the third were three times thinner than those of the second. On the average the fields of visual resolution decreased in size with increasing spatial frequency (decreasing bar width), and they were virtually identical whether the gratings had been imagined or observed. The imagery and the perceptual fields were also very similar in shape: resolu-

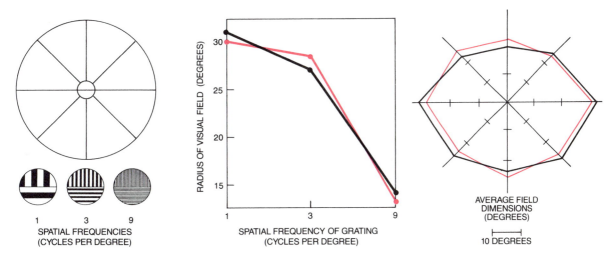

Figure 12.2 CONSTRAINTS on visual resolution were measured by three patterns (*bottom left*). Subjects projected their mental images of each pattern onto the center of a large display (*top left*), then indicated how far they could look away from their images along each of the eight lines on the display before they could no longer tell the two halves of the imagined patterns apart. The fields of visual resolution decreased with increasing spatial frequency, or decreasing bar width (*colored line, middle*). These fields were elongated horizontally and larger below the direction of gaze than above it (*colored shape, right*). Similar results (*black line, middle; black shape, right*) were obtained when the patterns were actually projected on the display.

tion decreased more slowly along the horizontal axis than along the vertical axis, as well as more slowly below the point of fixation than above it.

We then did a control experiment in which we showed a different group of subjects the original set of three disks and asked them to predict the image-resolution fields. Their predictions differed considerably from what we had observed, arguing against a trivial "guessing" explanation of our original findings.

We interpret the results as evidence that pattern discrimination in imagery is constrained in much the same way that it is in visual perception. We propose in addition that these mutual constraints are probably imposed at the pattern-processing levels of the visual system, where the properties of certain neural mechanisms may limit the ability to resolve small or narrowly spaced visual features. Kurtzman and I have done other experiments that are consistent with this result. We found no correspondence between judgments of images and judgments of objects involving differing amounts of visual contrast, or relative brightness, among features. These aspects of perception are thought to be constrained by more primitive kinds of neural processes operating below the levels at which pattern processing takes place.

Our image-resolution findings were based on mental images of flat, two-dimensional patterns. Mental imagery is typically three-dimensional, however; it depicts how objects look in depth as they are viewed from various vantages. When most people imagine their living room, for instance, they can mentally "see" that certain pieces of furniture are in front of others, depending on where in the living room they imagine themselves to be.

To investigate the three-dimensional properties of images, Steven Pinker and I asked subjects to form and mentally rotate images of a configuration of objects in space. When one actually looks at a three-dimensional configuration of objects from different perspectives, the objects are usually seen to shift their relative position in depth as the viewer moves or as the configuration is rotated. Recall, for example, times when you may have watched people riding on a merry-go-round. You probably noted that the people would appear to shift their locations in relation to your vantage as the merry-go-round turned, perhaps forming familiar two-dimensional patterns at certain moments in much the same way that a constellation of stars often forms flat, recog-

nizable patterns. In our experiments, which we did at Harvard, we were particularly interested in finding out whether similar kinds of patterns would appear to emerge when subjects imagined looking at a rotated configuration of objects. The results indicate striking similarities.

We asked our subjects first to learn the locations of four small plastic animals suspended at different heights in a transparent cylinder, and then to form mental images of them after they were removed (see Figure 12.3). We next rotated the empty cylinder 90 degrees and instructed the subjects to draw the imagined configuration as it now appeared from the new vantage. If they had imagined and rotated the animals with perfect accuracy as we rotated the cylinder, the animals would have seemed to form a parallelogram.

In every case the subjects' drawings revealed that their rotated mental images had depicted a pattern closely resembling the parallelogram, even though the appearance of the objects from the original viewing direction did not suggest that this particular geometric form would emerge. Curiously, there were small but systematic distortions in the drawings. The nature of the distortions suggested that the mental rotations had been less than perfectly accurate.

An explanation of these small distortions was suggested by another experiment, in which the subjects manually rotated the cylinder in order to align pairs of the imagined animals vertically. To our surprise we found that the subjects aligned the imagined animals by consistently rotating the cylinder less than was necessary when the animals were physically present. In other words, the subjects had mentally rotated their images ahead of their manual rotation of the cylinder. This tendency to advance an image ahead by small amounts accounted for the minor distortions we had found in our subjects' drawings of the emergent patterns. The experiment thus strengthened our contention that people can accurately imagine the visual perspectives offered by three-dimensional displays. Moreover, it enabled us to measure properties of mental images that naive subjects would not ordinarily expect.

Showing that subjects cannot guess the outcome of an imagery experiment does not, however, rule out the possibility that their performance could be based on unconscious knowledge about changes in the visual appearance of objects—knowledge that could indirectly influence judgments about images. One method for addressing this problem is

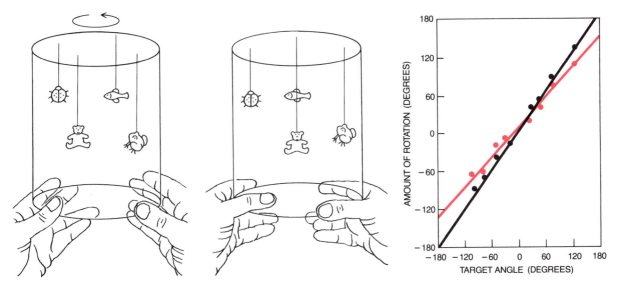

Figure 12.3 THREE-DIMENSIONAL PROPERTIES of mental images were explored. Subjects first learned the locations of four plastic animals suspended in a transparent cylinder and formed mental images of them. As the empty cylinder was rotated 90 degrees, the subjects rotated their mental images (*left*). Their drawings of the pattern were fairly accurate but showed small, systematic distortions. In a control experiment, to align pairs of the imagined animals vertically (*middle*), subjects rotated the cylinder manually by a consistently smaller amount (*colored line, right*) than they did in a test with the animals present (*black line, right*). The subjects had mentally rotated their images ahead of their manual rotation of the cylinder.

to have subjects imagine events so atypical or unnatural that the events could not have been previously experienced. If under these conditions behavioral responses obtained from imagery still correspond to those obtained from perception, the imagery performance could not be attributed to the influence of earlier perceptual experiences.

In a series of experiments I carried out at the Massachusetts Institute of Technology, I attempted to provide this kind of evidence for the functional value of imagery by considering the possible role images might play in prism adaptation. Optical prisms displace the apparent location of objects. A large body of research has shown that people quickly adapt to observing the world through such prisms provided they can move about and note their errors. When the prisms are removed following adaptation, people proceed to make errors of movement in the opposite direction, reflecting changes in their visual-motor coordination. My experiments demonstrated that prism adaptation can occur even when people point at a target and merely imagine they are making errors of movement like those typically induced by displacement prisms.

The subjects in my experiments wore special glasses containing optical prisms. I asked the sub-jects in one group to extend their right arms and point to a red marker positioned at eye level on a table in front of them. Owing to the effect of the prisms they at first pointed about five centimeters to the right of the marker. Since the prisms displace everything in the field of view, once the individuals had extended their arms they could see their errors and correct for them during a series of subsequent attempts (see Figure 12.4).

I measured and averaged the errors over consecutive groups of trials and then displayed the average error locations with three markers. The markers were for the use of a second group of subjects known as the imagery subjects. These subjects also wore the special glasses, but the area between them and the table holding the markers was covered by a board so that they could not see the fingers of their outstretched arms. I instructed the imagery subjects to point to the red marker while looking through the prisms and then to imagine they saw their pointing finger arrive under the appropriate error marker as soon as their arm was fully extended.

The error markers, in other words, ensured that the imagined errors would correspond to the average pointing errors made by the first group of subjects. I also included a third group of subjects as

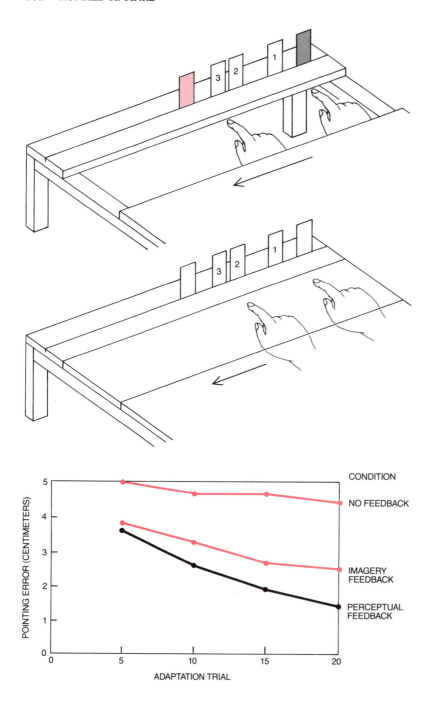

CONDITION

NO FEEDBACK

IMAGERY
FEEDBACK

PERCEPTUAL
FEEDBACK

Figure 12.4 PRISMS DISPLACE the apparent location of an object. Subjects wearing glasses containing such prisms were told to point to a target (*colored marker, top row*). They first pointed to the right of the marker (*gray marker*), but once they had extended their arms, they could see their fingers and correct for the error in successive attempts (*markers 1–3*). The markers were then used by a second group of subjects who wore the special glasses but could not see their fingers (*second row*). Their task was to imagine that they saw their pointing finger arrive under the appropriate error marker. Subjects in a control group pointed to the colored marker without being able to observe their errors. The graph (*bottom*) gives the results.

controls. The individuals in the control group pointed to the red marker without having the benefit of either observing their errors or being told to imagine them.

Only the subjects in the perception and imagery conditions showed a significant reduction in pointing error. Moreover, their rates of adaptation were similar. The results for pointing aftereffects, which take place when the glasses are removed, provide additional support for a functional equivalence between observed and imagined errors. Although the aftereffects in the imagery condition were smaller than those in the perception condition, the subjects in both groups pointed to the left of the red marker when normal viewing conditions were restored. I also found evidence of intermanual transfer: the subjects not only pointed to the left with their right hand (the "adapted" hand) but also pointed to the left with their left hand (the "unadapted" hand).

The findings have several implications. First, it is highly improbable that the subjects could have predicted the adaptation and transfer characteristics of prism-induced changes in their visual-motor coordination. It also seems unlikely that they could have had any related kinds of visual experiences providing them with unconscious knowledge of such effects. Second, the findings show that mental imagery can produce certain changes in visual-motor coordination that persist even after the images are no longer formed. They also suggest that the utilization of mental imagery to precipitate such changes may have important practical applications. Professional athletes, for example, often report they find it helpful to rehearse their performance mentally; in the light of these experiments it is reasonable to expect that the success of such techniques depends on the clarity and accuracy with which the performance is imagined.

The research findings I have discussed so far illustrate many ways mental images can correspond functionally to physically perceived objects and events. A question of greater practical significance is whether mental imagery can directly facilitate ongoing perceptual processes, assuming that a functional equivalence occurs. Given that similar constraints are imposed on visual resolution in imagery and perception, would it be possible, for instance, to see an object more quickly if an appropriate mental image of the object were formed in advance of its actual appearance?

As proposed some 10 years ago by Ulric Neisser and Lynn A. Cooper, then at Cornell, and Roger N. Shepard of Stanford University, the process of forming a mental image can serve a perceptual anticipatory function: it can prepare a person to receive information about imagined objects. Mental imagery may therefore enhance the perception of an object by causing the selective priming of appropriate neural mechanisms in the visual system. In other words, forming a mental image of an object might initiate certain neural events that are equiva-

lent to those occurring at the moment the object is seen, thereby facilitating the perceptual process.

If an object appears that is different from the one imagined, however, the formation of the image might interfere with the normal operation of the visual system. Suppose, for instance, that you are flying an airplane through a cloud. You might see the runway sooner if you were to imagine it in advance at its proper location. If, on the other hand, you imagined the runway at a different location, you might take longer to see it correctly than if you had not imagined it at all.

Some recent experiments I did at Stanford help to clarify the practical relation between image formation and object perception. In one of the experiments subjects indicated whether they saw either a horizontal bar or a vertical bar on a circular screen. These two alternative bars were known as target bars. I told the subjects to form, in advance, a mental image of an identically shaped bar oriented somewhere between the horizontal and the vertical, or to form no mental image. In each trial, therefore, one of the two alternative target bars was superposed on an imagined bar (in those cases where a bar was imagined). I recorded the reaction time for identifying the target bar as a function of the relative alignment between it and the imagined bar. The reaction times for the no-image trials served as a baseline measure.

The subjects made the quickest bar identifications when the imagined bars were closely aligned with the target bars, within a range of about 10 degrees. As the angle between the imagined and the target bars was increased to 45 degrees the identification time also increased. For angles greater than 45 degrees the time decreased once again. In other words, the maximum interference in identification took place when the bars had been imagined to lie exactly in between the two possible target orientations.

Why did the reaction times simply not increase in direct proportion to the degree of misalignment between the imagined and the target bars? One reason is that the subjects' selection of responses could have been based on a comparison between the mental image and the target. If the image matches the target, the response corresponding to the image orientation is quickly selected. If the image and the target differ by 90 degrees, the comparison indicates that the response opposite to the one corresponding to the image orientation is correct. If the imagined bar is in between the two target orientations, however, the comparison becomes confusing and the image interferes with the decision process.

A second experiment supports this explanation. In it I instructed the subjects to indicate as quickly as possible whether either of the two target bars appeared. In the previous experiment they had to distinguish between the two targets; in this case they only had to detect the presence of any target, without having to identify it. The results of this experiment clearly show that mental imagery did not affect simple detection judgments under those conditions. It seems, therefore, that even though image formation may influence the identification of visual patterns, it may not influence the more elementary process of simply detecting any stimulus change.

Additional experiments that Jennifer J. Freyd and I carried out at Stanford provide evidence for a kind of image facilitation that cannot be explained on the basis of response selection. In these experiments we studied the effects of forming a mental image that could serve as a helpful or unhelpful visual context for making difficult length discriminations. We presented our subjects with patterns consisting of two straight lines that formed a simple cross and asked them to indicate which line was longer. At the be-

ginning of certain trials we told the subjects to form an image of an outlined square, which if actually superposed on the center of the line pattern would have enhanced the small differences in the lengths of the lines. During other trials we told the subjects to form an image of an X (the endpoints of which corresponded to the four corners of the imagined square), which would presumably not have been as useful for making the discriminations (see Figure 12.5).

We found that forming a mental image of the helpful context pattern (the square) reduced the time needed to make the length discriminations compared with the time required when the unhelpful pattern (the X) was imagined or when subjects were not told to form images. Moreover, the effects were similar to those obtained when the same context patterns were actually presented.

We also found that subjects often chose to imagine the helpful context pattern when they were presented with positional cues they could use to imagine either pattern. Since the context patterns themselves could not have biased the selection of the two response alternatives, this type of image facilitation could not have resulted from an internal matching or response-selection process. Instead it may be due to a mental synthesis of real and imagined features at some higher level of the visual

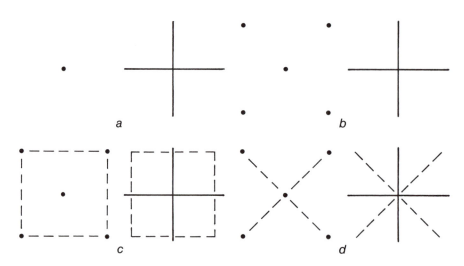

Figure 12.5 DISCRIMINATION TASK was assisted by mental imagery. Subjects were asked to determine whether a horizontal or a vertical line was the longer. In condition *a* the subjects looked at a fixation point and were then shown the two lines centered at that point. In *b* they were first shown four dots surrounding the fixation point. In *c* they were shown the same dots as in *b* and were asked to form a mental image of a square frame connecting them. In *d* they were asked to form an image of an X through the four dots. The greatest facilitation in the length-discrimination judgments came from imagining the square frame in advance.

system—where the addition of context information can enhance differences among objects that are being compared.

In each of the techniques described up to this point experimental subjects were told explicitly to form some kind of mental image. A possible difficulty with this procedure is that it may encourage the subjects to try to perform as they would in a corresponding perceptual task, thinking that is what they are supposed to do. Although the problem can be largely avoided by attempting to measure subtle or unexpected perceptual effects, an even better way is to show that images can be formed spontaneously for some specific purpose even when no imagery instructions of any kind are given.

The importance of these considerations follows from early studies done by Kosslyn and Pinker on mental-image scanning. They asked subjects to inspect a configuration of objects (such as landmark items drawn on a map), form a mental image of the configuration and "focus in" on one of the objects. The investigators then named a second object and told the subjects to mentally scan along a direct path from the first object to the second. Kosslyn and Pinker consistently found that the time required to complete the mental-image scanning was directly proportional to the original physical distance between the objects, and they therefore concluded that mental images preserve the spatial characteristics of a physical display.

Their findings have been criticized because it would not be hard for experimental subjects to figure out that greater distances should require longer

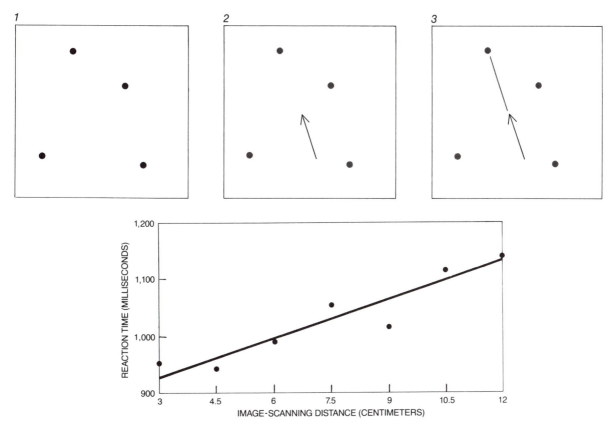

Figure 12.6 MENTAL IMAGES can be exploited to scan patterns. Subjects were first shown a dot pattern (1) and then an arrow in the same field. Their task was to determine if the arrow was pointing to any of the previously seen dots. They reported that in order to make the judgment they had to generate an image of the dot pattern (2) and then scan the image along the direction indicated by the arrow to see if any of the dots would be intercepted (3). The graph shows that the larger the distance between dots and arrows was, the longer it took a subject to make the judgment. The dependence of reaction time on distance provides evidence for a process of image scanning.

scanning times. Pinker and I have since developed a task that seems to avoid this problem by requiring a subject to form mental images and scan them without explicit directions to do so. After they had inspected a dot pattern, our subjects were shown an arrow and were asked to indicate whether it pointed at any of the previously seen dots. We had predicted that, in order to see if any of the dots would be intercepted, the subjects would have to scan a men-

tal image of the pattern along the direction specified by the arrow (see Figure 12.6).

The experiment turned out to be successful. The decision times increased linearly as distance along the scan path between the arrows and the dots increased. Moreover, nearly all the subjects reported that in order to perform the task they had to form and scan a mental image of the dot pattern. We thus showed that mental-image scanning can be useful

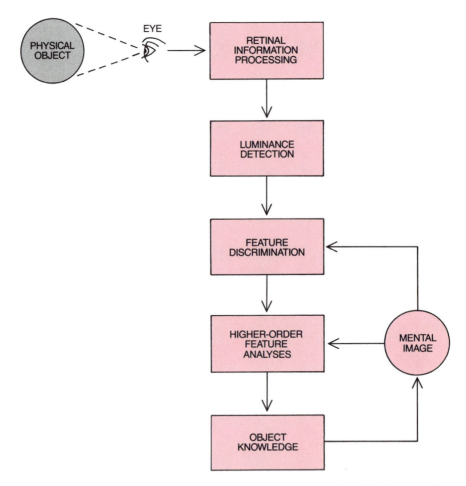

Figure 12.7 MENTAL IMAGERY may influence visual perception. Perception of an object is a result of neural activation within a sequence of information-processing stages in the visual system, beginning at the retinal level (*top*). Image formation is determined by the knowledge a person has about the features of the object; presumably it occurs at the very highest levels. Once formed, an image may affect neural mechanisms, at intermediate visual levels, that are responsible for feature discrimination and other more complex types of analyses, perhaps modifying perception of the object. Mental imagery probably does not influence visual levels below those concerned with feature discrimination.

whenever it is necessary to anticipate the consequences of moving along a particular path from a given starting point.

Suppose you were trying to figure out where a billiard ball would come to rest on a billiard table after you had aimed it in a certain direction. Even if you could not actually roll the ball across the table or determine the answer mathematically, you could still imagine what would happen by mentally following the motion of the ball and its reflections off the cushions. Cooper and Shepard have reported related findings for the imagined consequences of rotating objects [see "Turning Something Over in the Mind," by Lynn A. Cooper and Roger N. Shepard; SCIENTIFIC AMERICAN, December, 1984].

In the light of these studies it seems reasonable to propose that whenever imagery and perception share common neural mechanisms in the visual system, imagery could facilitate the perceptual processes those mechanisms support. One should therefore seek to determine the lowest visual levels at which such mechanisms may be shared. If visual pattern perception, for instance, is conceived of as involving an orderly sequence of information-processing stages ranging from the lowest to the highest levels of the visual system, one might begin by trying to discover how far down in this sequence image formation can influence the underlying mechanisms (see Figure 12.7).

Starting at the very lowest, or retinal, level, where the most primitive types of information-processing mechanisms are found, one would not expect mental imagery to have much effect. Nor would mental imagery be expected to alter information processing at precortical levels, where mechanisms are responsible for detecting changes in brightness or contrast. Only at the somewhat higher levels responsible for pattern discrimination (as in the visual cortex) does one begin to find evidence that mental images can influence perception. At still higher levels the evidence is strong that imagery can influence perception.

Finally, at the very highest levels one may assume that perceptual processes interact with more abstract processes having to do with knowledge about and understanding of physical objects. Here it is helpful to make a distinction between the form and the function of a mental image. When a person decides to create a mental image of a particular object, the kind of image that can be fashioned depends on the knowledge the person has about the object, such as its size, color and shape. Then once the image is formed it can begin to function in some respects like the object itself, bringing about the activation of certain types of neural mechanisms at lower levels in the visual system. Accordingly, whatever constraints such mechanisms put on the quality of one's perception of the object are also placed on the quality of one's mental imagery. In this way mental images may come to acquire visual characteristics and may serve to modify perception itself.

The Authors

DAVID H. HUBEL and TORSTEN N. WIESEL ("Brain Mechanisms of Vision") are neurobiologists. Hubel is the John Franklin Enders University Professor and professor of neurobiology at Harvard Medical School. Born in Windsor, Ontario, he received his B.Sc. and M.D. degrees from McGill University. He has been at Harvard Medical School conducting research in neurobiology since 1960. Wiesel is the Vincent and Brooke Astor Professor and head of the Laboratory of Neurobiology at Rockefeller University. Born in Sweden, he obtained his M.D. in 1954 at the Karolinska Institute in Stockholm. Hubel and Wiesel have collaborated on studies of the mammalian visual system for nearly 20 years.

OLGA EIZNER FAVREAU and MICHAEL C. CORBALLIS ("Negative Aftereffects in Visual Perception") are, respectively, professor of psychology at the University of Montreal and professor of psychology at the University of Auckland, Auckland, New Zealand. Favreau earned her Ph.D. at McGill in 1973 and is interested in the field of visual perception. Corballis received his Ph.D. in psychology from McGill in 1965. He is interested in most aspects of cognitive neuropsychology.

EDWIN H. LAND ("The Retinex Theory of Color Vision") is president and director of research at The Rowland Institute for Science in Cambridge, Massachusetts. Land has received 15 honorary degrees, has held visiting academic appointments at Harvard and is currently Visiting Institute Professor at the Massachusetts Institute of Technology. In 1967 he received the National Medal of Science, and in 1977, on the occasion of his 500th U.S. patent, he was elected to the National Inventors Hall of Fame. Land currently has 537 patents.

ALAN L. GILCHRIST ("The Perception of Surface Blacks and Whites") is associate professor of psychology at the State University of New York at Stony Brook. He grew up in the Pacific Northwest and received his bachelor's degree from Portland State College. He then came east to do graduate work at the Institute for Cognitive Studies at Rutgers University, obtaining his Ph.D. there in 1975.

TOMASO POGGIO ("Vision by Man and Machine") is the Uncas and Helen Whitaker Professor in the Department of Brain and Cognitive Science and a member of the Artificial Intelligence Lab at MIT. He received his Ph.D. in theoretical physics at the University of Genoa. Poggio collaborated with the late David Marr of MIT on the computational approach to vision and more recently has been trying to understand the information-processing mechanism of the brain and its basis in the biophysical properties of nerve cells.

ANNE TREISMAN ("Features and Objects in Visual Processing") is professor of psychology at the University of California at Berkeley. She received her undergraduate education at the University of Cambridge and her graduate training at the University of Oxford. She was elected a member of the Royal Society of London in 1989.

IRVIN ROCK ("The Perception of Disoriented Figures") is adjunct professor in the Department of Psychology at the University of California at Berkeley. He received his Ph.D. from the New School for Social Research in 1952. His major interest is in the field of visual perception.

VILAYANUR S. RAMACHANDRAN ("Perceiving Shape from Shading" and "The Perception of Apparent Motion," coauthor) is professor of psychology at the University of California, San Diego, and has a joint appointment as a visiting associate in biology at the California Institute of Technology. He obtained an M.D. at the University of Madras in 1974 and a Ph.D. in neurophysiology from the University of Cambridge in 1978. His current research goal is to find physiological mechanisms underlying the perceptual effects described in the chapter.

VILAYANUR S. RAMACHANDRAN and STUART M. ANSTIS ("The Perception of Apparent Motion"). Anstis is professor of psychology at York University in Toronto. He got an M.A. and a Ph.D. from the University of Cambridge, where he remained for two more years as a postdoctoral fellow. He taught at the University of Bristol before moving to York. Notes on Ramachandran appear in the preceding biography.

GAETANO KANIZSA ("Subjective Contours") is professor of psychology at the University of Trieste. He received his doctorate in psychology from the University of Padua. Since then he has dedicated himself "to the phenomenology of visual perception and thought processes." He carried on his work in Florence and Milan before returning to his native city of Trieste in 1953 to take up his present post.

BARBARA GILLAM ("Geometrical Illusions") is chair person of the department of psychology at the University of New South Wales in Australia, where she conducts research in visual perception and binocular vision. She received her Ph.D. for her work on binocular vision from the Australian National University. She is interested in various topics in the field of perception.

RONALD A. FINKE ("Mental Imagery and the Visual System") is associate professor at Texas A&M University. He earned his doctorate in psychology at the Massachusetts Institute of Technology in 1979. He is interested in distortions in visual memory and the psychology of belief in paranormal phenomena.

Bibliographies

1. Brain Mechanisms of Vision

Mountcastle, V. B. 1957. Modality and topographic properties of single neurons of cat's somatic sensory cortex. *The Journal of Neurophysiology* 20(4) (July): 408–434.

Hubel, D. H., and T. N. Wiesel. 1968. Receptive fields and functional architecture of monkey striate cortex. *The Journal of Physiology* 195(2) (November): 215–244.

Hubel, D. H., and T. N. Wiesel. 1977. Ferrier lecture: Functional architecture of macaque monkey visual cortex. *Proceedings of the Royal Society of London, Series B* 198:1–59.

Hubel, D. H., T. N. Wiesel and M. P. Stryker. 1978. Anatomical demonstration of orientation columns in macaque monkey. *The Journal of Comparative Neurology* 177(3) (February 1): 361–379.

Hubel, D. H. 1982. Exploration of the primary visual cortex 1955–1978. *Nature* 299:515–524.

Hubel, D. H. 1987. *Eye, Brain, and Vision.* W. H. Freeman and Company.

2. Negative Aftereffects in Visual Perception

Over, R. 1971. Comparison of normalization theory and neural enhancement explanation of negative aftereffects. *Psychological Bulletin* 75(4) (April): 225–243.

Carterette, E. C., and M. P. Friedman, eds. 1973. *Handbook of perception,* vol. I: *Historical and philosophical roots of perception.* Academic Press.

Kaufman, L. 1974. *Sight and mind: An introduction to visual perception.* Oxford University Press.

Anstis, S. M. 1975. What does visual perception tell us about visual coding? In *Handbook of Psychobiology,* eds. M. S. Gazzaniga and C. Blakemore. Academic Press.

Skowko, D., B. N. Timney, T. A. Gentry and R. B. Morant. 1975. McCollough effects: Experimental findings and theoretical accounts. *Psychological Bulletin* 82(4) (July): 497–510.

3. The Retinex Theory of Color Vision

Land, E. H. 1959. Color vision and the natural image: Part I. *Proceedings of the National Academy of Sciences* 45(1) (January): 115–129.

Land, E. H. 1959. Color vision and the natural image: Part II. *Proceedings of the National Academy of Sciences* 45(4) (April): 636–644.

McCann, J. J., and J. L. Benton. 1969. Interaction of the long-wave cones and the rods to produce color sensations. *Journal of the Optical Society of America* 59(1) (January): 103–107.

Land, E. H., and J. J. McCann. 1971. Lightness and retinex theory. *Journal of the Optical Society of America* 61(1) (January): 1–11.

Land, E. H. 1983. Recent advances in retinex theory and some implications for cortical computation: Color vision and the natural image. *Proceedings of the National Academy of Science* 80 (August): 5163–5169.

Land, E. H. 1986. An alternative technique for the computation of the designator in the retinex theory of color vision. *Proceedings of the National Academy of Science* 83 (May): 3078–3080.

4. The Perception of Surface Blacks and Whites

Yarbus, A. L. 1967. Eye movements and vision. Trans., B. Haigh. Plenum Press.

Walraven, J. 1976. Discounting the background—the missing link in the explanation of chromatic induction. *Vision Research* 16:289–295.

Gilchrist, A. L. 1977. Perceived lightness depends on perceived spatial arrangement. *Science* 195(4274) (January 14): 185–187.

Land, E. H. 1977. The retinex theory of color vision. *Scientific American* 237(6) (December): 108–128.

5. Vision By Man and Machine

Winston, P. H. 1977. *Artificial intelligence.* Addison-Wesley Publishing Co.

Marr, D., and T. Poggio. 1979. A computational theory of human stereo vision. *Proceedings of the Royal*

Society of London, Series B 204(1156) (May 23): 301–328.

Grimison, W. E. L. 1981. *From images to surfaces: A computational study of the human early visual system.* The MIT Press.

Reichardt, W. E., and T. Poggio, eds. 1981. *Theoretical approaches in neurobiology.* The MIT Press.

Nishihara, H. K. 1981. Intensity, visible-surface, and volumetric representations. *Artificial Intelligence* 17(1–3) (August): 265–284.

Marr, D. 1982. *Vision.* W. H. Freeman and Company.

Poggio, T., E. B. Gamble and J. J. Little. 1988. Parallel integration of vision modules. *Science* 242 (October 21): 337–484.

6. Features and Objects in Visual Processing

Frisby, P. 1980. *Seeing: Illusion, brain, and mind.* Oxford University Press.

Rock, I. 1984. *Perception.* Scientific American Books, Inc. See Chapter 5. Form and organization.

Treisman, A. 1986. Properties, parts and objects. *Handbook of Perception and Performance*, Vol. 2, eds., K. Boff, L. Kaufman and J. Thomas. John Wiley & Sons, Inc.

Treisman, A. 1988. Features and objects: The fourteenth Bartlett memorial lecture. *Journal of Experimental Psychology* 140A:201–237.

Treisman, A., and S. Gormican. 1988. Feature analysis in early vision: Evidence from search asymmetries. *Psychological Review* 95:15–48.

7. The Perception of Disoriented Figures

Dearborn, G. V. N. 1899. Recognition under objective reversal. *Psychological Review* 6(4) (July): 395–406.

Mach, E. 1959. *The analysis of sensations and the relation of the physical to the psychical.* C. M. Williams, trans. Dover Publications, Inc.

Howard, I. P., and W. B. Templeton. 1966. Orientation and shape I and II. In *Human Spatial Orientation.* John Wiley & Sons, Inc.

Goldmeier, E. 1972. Similarity in visually perceived forms. *Psychological Issues* 8(1) Monograph 29.

Rock, I. 1974. *Orientation and form.* Academic Press.

8. Perceiving Shape from Shading

Yonas, A., M. Kuskowski and S. Sternfels. 1979. The role of frames of reference in the development of responsiveness to shading. *Child Development* 50(2) (June): 495–500.

Todd, J. T., and E. Mingolla. 1983. Perception of surface curvature and direction of illumination from patterns of illumination from patterns of shading. *Journal of Experimental Psychology: Human Perception and Performance* 9(4) (August): 583–595.

Ramachandran, V. S. 1988. Perception of shape from shading. *Nature* 331(6152) (January 14): 133–166.

9. The Perception of Apparent Motion

Ramachandran, V. S., V. M. Rao and T. R. Vidyasagar. 1973. Apparent movement with "subjective" contours. *Vision Research* 13 (July): 1399–1410.

Anstis, S. M. 1978. Apparent motion. *Handbook of Sensory Physiology*, Vol. 8, eds. R. Held, H. Leibowitz and H. L. Teuber. Springer-Verlag.

Ramachandran, V. S., and S. M. Anstis. 1983. Perceptual organization in moving patterns. *Nature* 304(5926) (August 11): 529–531.

10. Subjective Contours

Lawson, R. B., and W. L. Gulick, 1967. Stereopsis and anomalous contour. *Vision Research* 7 (March): 271–297.

Pastore, N. 1971. *Selective history of theories of visual perception: 1650–1950.* Oxford University Press.

Stadler, M., and J. Dieker. 1972. Untersuchungen zum problem virtueller konturen in der visuellen wahrnehmung. *Zeitschrift für experimentelle und angewandte Psychologie* 19(2):325–350.

Coren, S. 1972. Subjective contours and apparent depth. *Psychological Review* 79(4) (July): 359–367.

Gregory, R. L. 1972. Cognitive contours. *Nature* 238(5358) (July 7): 51–52.

Kanizsa, G. 1974. Contours without gradients or cognitive contours? *Italian Journal of Psychology* 1(1) (April): 93–112.

Petry, S., and G. Meyer, eds. 1987. *The perception of illusory contours.* Springer-Verlag.

11. Geometrical Illusions

Gillam, B. 1971. A depth processing theory of the Poggendorff illusion. *Perception and Psychophysics* 10(4A):211–216.

Robinson, J. O. 1972. *The psychology of visual illusion.* Hutchinson University Library.

Gregory, R. L., and E. H. Gombrich, eds. 1973. *Illusion in nature and art.* Charles Scribner's Sons.

Coren, S., and J. S. Girgus. 1978. Seeing is deceiving: *The psychology of visual illusions.* Laurence Erlbaum Associates.

12. Mental Imagery and the Visual System

Kosslyn, S. M. 1980. *Image and mind.* Harvard University Press.

Finke, R. A. 1980. Levels of equivalence in imagery and perception. *Psychological Review* 87(2) (March): 113–132.

Pinker, S. 1980. Mental imagery and the third dimension. *Journal of Experimental Psychology: General* 109(3) (September): 354–371.

Sources of the Photographs

1. David H. Hubel and Torsten N. Wiesel: Figures 1.2, 1.3, 1.5, 1.10, 1.11, 1.13, 1.14, 1.15, 1.19

3. Julius J. Scarpetti: Figures 3.1, 3.2, 3.5, 3.16, 3.19

4. Alan L. Gilchrist: Figures 4.4, 4.5

5. Robert J. Woodham: Figures 5.1 (top), 5.7 (left)
   W. Eric L. Grimson: Figure 5.1 (bottom)
   H. Keith Nishihara: Figures 5.2, 5.6
   Massachusetts Institute of Technology: Figure 5.7 (right)

6. Jon Brenneis: Figure 6.1

7. Wide World Photos: Figure 7.1

8. Vilayanur S. Ramachandran: Figure 8.1
   George V. Kelvin: Figures 8.2, 8.3, 8.4, 8.5, 8.7, 8.8, 8.9, 8.10

9. The Granger Collection: Figure 9.1
   Vilayanur S. Ramachandran and Patrick Cavanagh: Figure 9.9

10. Stephen Cass: Figure 12.1

INDEX

Page numbers in *italics* indicate illustrations.